Measuring Medical Practice

Statistics for the Physician

W9-BEX-686

American Medical Association Division of Health Policy and Program Evaluation

Foreword

Statistics has always played an important role in medicine. All physicians, whether they are involved in teaching, research, administration, management, or patient care, have traditionally found statistics to be an important tool in their professional lives.

Recently, however, statistics has taken on a significantly greater role, primarily in the area of medical review. In an era of continuing concerns over costs of health care, and mounting efforts to assess and evaluate the quality of care, statistics is increasingly being used in health care assessment.

Increasingly, physicians are being confronted with, and often asked to account for, statistical reports of their practice patterns. These include rate of hospital admissions, average length of hospital stays, use of medical resources, and patient outcomes.

While much of this review may be helpful, this increased emphasis on statistical review poses difficult problems for the practicing physician. The interpretation of statistical reports often requires the physician to possess a level of sophistication that his training did not provide. Typically concerned with the diagnosis and treatment of the individual patient, the physician may find statistical methodologies—with their emphasis on the characteristics of a group—alien to his way of thinking about medical care. This may help to account for the difficulty some physicians have in interpreting statistics.

Finally, there is an ever-present danger that statistical methods may be used incorrectly or inappropriately, or even misused.

It is thus increasingly important that physicians be equipped with fundamental information about the science of statistics. Only a physician knowledgeable about statistics will be able to respond effectively to the evolving environment of medical review. Only by understanding statistics will physicians be able to continue their role as advocates for the individual patient.

The purpose of this booklet, then, is to provide physicians with a basic understanding of statistics, and particularly of what statistics should and should not be asked to do. Fundamental concepts and principles in statistics are presented in a format designed for both reading and reference, with a glossary of key terms at the end of the document; mathematics is kept to a minimum in order to increase readability. The booklet discusses some of the more important applications of statistics in medicine, and describes some of the statistical methods that may properly be employed in clinical situations. In the final section, the booklet discusses special problems that confront physicians today: area-to-area variations in statistics pertaining to the delivery of health care, the release of hospital mortality data, utilization review, quality assurance, and the activities of peer review organizations (PROs).

This booklet will not make its readers into practicing biostatisticians. But it will, it is hoped, make them more critical consumers, better able to evaluate statistical information and raise pertinent questions about the use (and misuse) of statistics in medicine.

James H. Sammons, M.D.
Executive Vice President

November 1987

Acknowledgments

The AMA wishes to acknowledge the significant contributions made by a number of individuals in development and production of this monograph. Jerald R. Schenken, M.D., Barry S. Eisenberg and Jack A. Moshman, Ph.D. were largely responsible for conceptualization of the document and organization of the content. Doris L. Konicki made significant content and editorial contributions. The AMA Center for Health Policy Research contributed substantial information and data for the section on Hospital Mortality Data. Others who provided invaluable assistance included: Christopher A. Damon, Kathy Kaye and Diana C. Lemons.

Contents

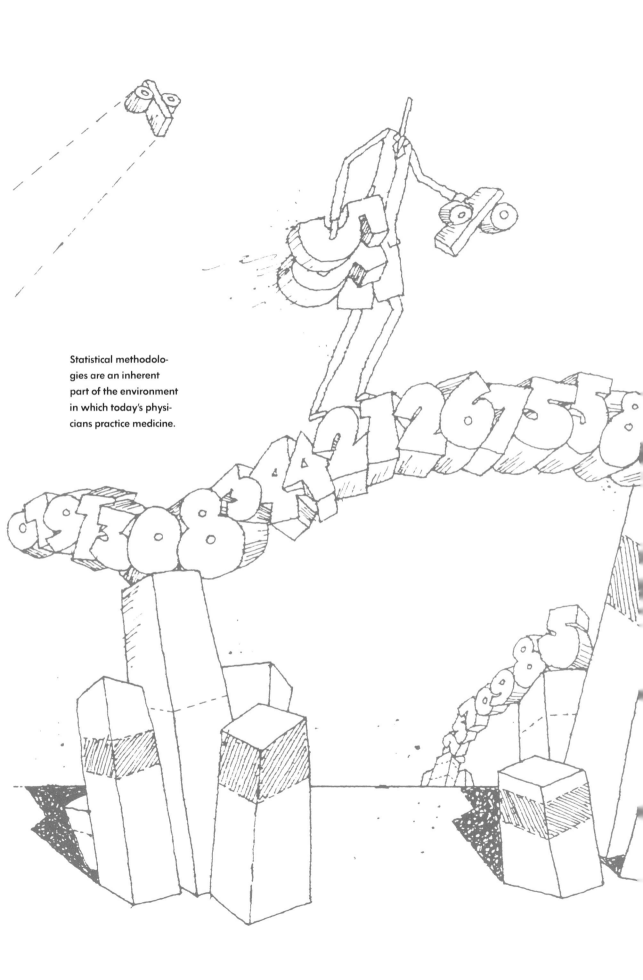

Statistical methodologies are an inherent part of the environment in which today's physicians practice medicine.

Introduction

A patient visits his physician for a physical examination and, in the course of that examination, is given a blood pressure reading.

The physician determines that this blood pressure reading is "high."

How was that determination made? "Clinical judgment," most physicians would resoundingly reply.

That would be an appropriate answer. Yet, what is clinical judgment? The physician's years of training and experience certainly play an important part, as does his intimate understanding of this patient's unique situation.

Nonetheless, the chances are that the physician also had some help from statistics.

For instance, the physician probably compared the patient's blood pressure reading to a range he knew to be "normal"—that is, a range of readings typical for a large percentage of the population. The process whereby this numerical information was collected, and the determination of what constitutes a "normal" range—all that is part of the science of statistics.

The physician may also have applied knowledge of the likelihood, or probability, that someone with a blood pressure reading in this patient's range will at some point in his life experience adverse health effects. This calculation of probability—even if the physician never actually computed it—is fundamentally statistical in nature.

What's more, the physician's choice of therapy for this patient will almost certainly be influenced by statistics. Typically, the efficacy of any new therapy is measured in statistical terms—often by comparison with some other accepted therapy, although in some cases the measurement is made in terms of some defined criterion of success, such as the ability of the patient to resume daily life or the length of time before the apparent remission of any symptoms. Regardless, a scientific evaluation of a new therapy almost invariably is made using statistics.

Finally, statistics are typically used in assessing the performance of individual physicians. Thus this physician's choice of tests and treatment might, at some point, be evaluated by comparison with a statistical analysis of what other physicians have done under similar circumstances.

In short, physicians use statistics all the time. Statistics are used in the consulting room, in the evaluation of laboratory tests, and in the review of research as reported in the medical literature. Statistical methodologies are an inherent part of the environment in which today's physicians practice medicine.

What is Statistics?   Statistics is the mathematical study of the behavior of groups. As a mathematical science, it has its own language, literature, and scientific notation.

Yet there need be nothing inherently difficult about the study of statistics. For statistics can be thought of, simply, as a quantified form of common sense.

Statistics provides the mathematical underpinning for mental processes that many people undertake informally every day—gathering information about groups, expressing that information in a compact way, and drawing inferences about how members of a group will behave, based on information about all or part of the group.

The composition of the group—also known as a *population* or *universe*—scarcely matters: The group may be made up of individuals, cases, events, or almost any other entities. Statistics works equally well for many different types of groups.

For statistical purposes, it is important, however, that the group have well-defined, consistent boundaries separating those who are in the group from those who are not. For instance, a group might consist of "all patients who have seen Doctor X during his career," or "all cases of influenza in the United States in the 1960s," or "all deaths in Cook County, Ill., in 1986." On the other hand, a group defined as, simply, "some patients" or "some illnesses" or "some deaths" would not be sufficiently well-defined for statistical purposes.

The science of statistics is divided into two branches, each of which approaches the study of groups in a slightly different way:

Descriptive statistics collects, compiles, summarizes, and presents data about an entire group. (Such data are sometimes known as a *complete census.*) The purpose of descriptive statistics is to represent a large mass of information with a few numbers, enabling the user to grasp essential features of the group in a relatively compact way.

Inferential statistics draws or rejects inferences about a group or its members, based on data from a sample representing that group. Sometimes this means that one studies the sample group, then draws inferences about the characteristics of the group as a whole. In other instances, inferential statistics may be used to formulate a hypothesis about the whole group, then test this hypothesis by studying the sample population.

Schools of Thought

There are two major schools of thought or approaches to statistical analysis: the classical approach and the Bayesian approach. Classical statistics, as described in this monograph, bases its inferences and estimates on the data collected or examined for analysis. Also termed the "frequentist" school, classical statisticians take advantage of all prior knowledge to design a study and interpret the findings, but the analysis is based solely on the collected information. The "Bayesian" school, named after the Rev. Thomas Bayes, an 18th century British clergyman, seeks to take advantage of prior knowledge in the interpretation and analysis itself and by doing so results may be adjusted accordingly.

Most available textbooks and applications in the literature reflect a classical approach. Bayesian statistics, reflects more recent research much of which is in the area of medical science. Both schools of thought have much to recommend. In many common applications, comparable results are obtained regardless of the approach. This booklet follows a classical approach because, currently, the reader is more apt to encounter this school of thought in practice and in most of the reference works likely to be consulted for further information and background. However, an awareness of Bayesian statistics may prove helpful in some instances.

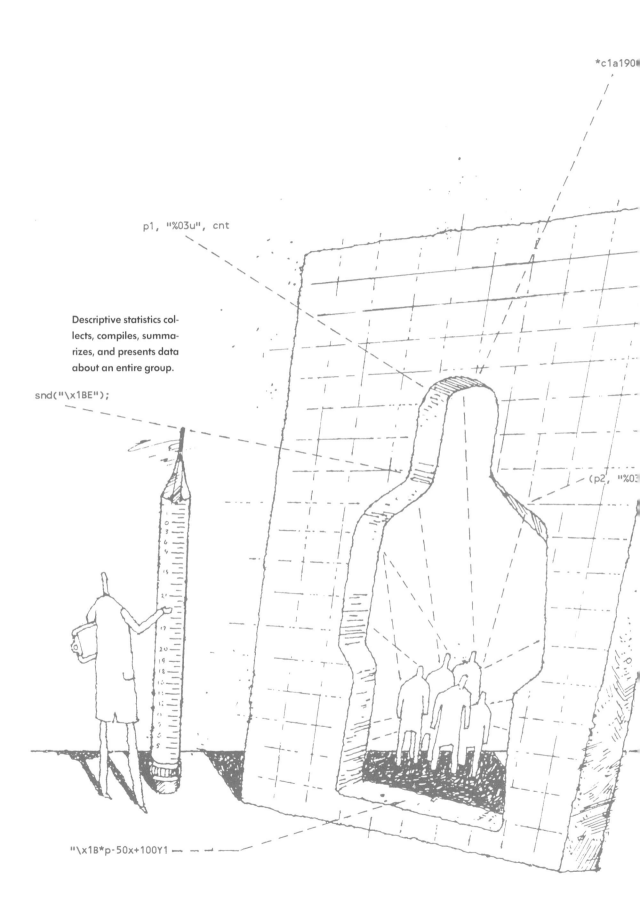

*c1a190

p1, "%03u", cnt

Descriptive statistics collects, compiles, summa-
rizes, and presents data
about an entire group.

snd("\x1BE");

(p2, "%0

"\x1B*p-50x+100Y1

Descriptive Statistics

Descriptive statistics collects, compiles, summarizes, and presents data about an entire group. Its purpose is to represent a large mass of information with a few numbers, enabling the user to grasp essential features of the group in a relatively compact way.

Examples of descriptive statistics abound in our society. A very simple one, published in the newspapers every day, is the batting average of baseball players. To calculate a batting average, we count every time the player has had an official "at bat" and find the proportion of the times he was at bat that he had a hit. The result is a concise way of describing the entire group of appearances the player has made at the plate during a specific period or of a specific type—e.g., this season, in his lifetime, or against left-handed pitchers.

In summarizing information about populations, people frequently talk about "averages." But what do we mean by *average?*

In statistics, an *average* is regarded as a measure of central tendency within a population. It can be calculated in any of several ways: as an *arithmetic mean,* as a *median,* or as a *mode.* Each of these measures offers certain advantages and disadvantages, depending on the situation.

To illustrate these measures, consider the following 25 numbers—which might represent, for example, the ages of a group of patients. Ranked in order of size, they are:

16	20	22	24	25
18	21	23	24	26
19	21	23	24	27
19	21	24	25	79
20	22	24	25	81

What is the average age of this group?

Arithmetic Mean

When people say *average,* they most often are referring to what statisticians call the *arithmetic mean.* It is obtained by adding the values for all members of the group and dividing by the total number of members. The arithmetic mean of the numbers listed above is obtained by adding up all the values and dividing by 25. The arithmetic mean (what many people would call the "average age" of the group) is thus 26.92. Notably, if every value on the list above were replaced by 26.92, the sum of all ages would remain the same.

Among the advantages of the arithmetic mean is that is easy to compute. But it does have a potential disadvantage: it is strongly affected by extreme numbers.

For example, the list above includes two values that are very large in comparison to the rest of the list: 79 and 81. If they were excluded and the mean were recalculated—513 divided by 23—the mean would be 22.30. Inclusion of these large values made the arithmetic mean considerably larger than it would otherwise have been. An arithmetic mean can produce a misleading impression of a group, particularly if the group contains some extreme values.

Median

Another type of average, or measure of central tendency, is the *median*. It is that number which is exceeded by half of the values in the group and is itself larger than the other half of the values. In the example above, since the ages are already listed in order of their size, it's relatively easy to obtain the median: It's the middle number—in a list of 25 names, the 13th. The median is 23.

What if there were an even number of values in the group? The convention in statistics is to take the arithmetic mean of the two middle values as the median.

The median is employed in many situations because, unlike the arithmetic mean, it is not affected by extreme values. Data that typically contain extreme numbers, such as annual income, are frequently described by the median.

Mode

The *mode*, another measure of central tendency, is the value or values found most frequently in the group. To obtain the mode, look for repetitions: In the list above, the value 24 appears on the list more often than does any of the other values.

What would we do if some other number appeared just as often as did 24? That would not be a problem, as a group can have more than one mode.

Like the median, the mode is not affected by the presence of extremely large or extremely small values. It can be extremely useful in certain situations: Off-the-shelf models of medical prosthetics are designed based on modal measurements, for example.

Measures of Variation

No measure of central tendency is a complete picture of a given group. Mean, median, or mode—none of these measures tells us whether all the values for the group are clustered close together about the measure of central tendency or whether they are widely dispersed.

Thus, to complete the picture of the "average" in a group, we need some statement of the degree of variation characteristic of the data. There is more than one way to state this variation.

Range

The simplest, but crudest, is the *range*—the difference between the largest and smallest value. In the example given above, the range is 65, the difference between 81 and 16.

Standard Deviation

The measure most widely used is the *standard deviation,* often symbolized by the symbol *s,* sometimes by the Greek lower case sigma (σ). To obtain the standard deviation, we perform the following calculation:

1. Square the difference between each value and the arithmetic mean, often symbolized by $(x_i - \overline{x})^2$.

2. Sum the squares.

3. Divide the sum by the number of data items, a quantity often symbolized by *n*.

4. Take the square root of this average.

The standard deviation of the data above is 15.87. If the two extreme values, 79 and 81, were eliminated, the standard deviation of the remaining 23 observations would be reduced to 2.71.

Mathematically, the formula for computing a standard deviation looks like this:

$$s = \sqrt{\frac{\Sigma(x_i - \overline{x})^2}{n}}$$

The formula may also be shown in this fashion, which is mathematically equivalent to the formula just given:

$$s = \sqrt{\frac{n\Sigma x_i^2 - (\Sigma x_i)^2}{n^2}}$$

In these formulae, the symbol x stands for a measured quantity; the subscript allows us to distinguish between measured quantities when there are more than one. Thus, in our example, x_1, x_2 and x_3 stand for 16, 18, 19, and so on. The symbol x_i refers to x with the subscript successively replaced by 1, 2, 3, and so on to the end of the sequence. The capital letter sigma, Σ, refers to the sum of all the x values.

Most of us use descriptive statistics every day—typically, however, without realizing that the concepts we are referring to are actually statistical in nature. Measures of central tendency are among the most frequently used. But certain other concepts in descriptive statistics also crop up quite frequently.

Total Count

Perhaps the simplest is the *total count*—for instance, the number of people in the United States. The number of physicians graduated from U.S. medical schools is another total count, as is the number of first-year students in U.S. medical schools. In each of the last two cases, the total count is simply derived from a complete enumeration of the class size in each of the medical schools.

Proportions

A *proportion* is that part of the total population whose elements possess some specified characteristic. Each element has or does not have the characteristic. The National Mortality Tables published by the National Center for Health Statistics provide examples of proportions, representing the proportion of all deaths occurring from specific causes, assuming the accuracy of the reported cause of death on the death certificate.

Percentiles

Percentiles, which are values dividing the corresponding data of a group, are also concepts derived from descriptive statistics. The 35th percentile, for example, is that value which divides the population so that 35 percent of the elements are less than the value and 65 percent are greater; the 83rd percentile designates an 83-17 split. (The median is actually a special case of a percentile: it is the 50th percentile.) Frequently, the 25th and 75th percentiles are termed the *first* and *third quartiles*. (The little used term *second quartile* refers to the median.)

Statistics, particularly descriptive statistics, are frequently represented by means of charts or graphs. Some of the more common ones include pie charts, bar charts, line graphs, and time series.

An example of a simple, easily comprehended, yet graphically striking chart is the bar chart in Figure 1, which shows the 1978 distribution of Medicare beneficiaries in terms of amount reimbursed per person and the corresponding total Medicare expenditures. The chart allows us to make a relatively easy comparison between the distribution of Medicare beneficiaries and the distribution of expenditures. From this we see, for example, that 61 percent of the persons served in 1978 received less than $500 each, and these 61 percent received only 5.4 percent of funds expended. At the other extreme, fewer than 15 percent of the people accounted for more than 70 percent of expenditures.

Figure 1. Percent Distribution of Aged Persons Served and Amounts Reimbursed Under Hospital Insurance and/or Supplementary Medical Insurance by Amounts Reimbursed, 1978

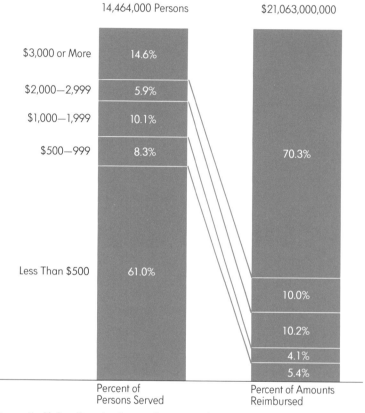

Source: Health Care Financing Program Statistics, Medicare Summary, 1982

An important consideration in the use of any chart or graph is that the scale employed not give a misleading impression of the data. Sometimes this happens because the data to be illustrated have not been selected appropriately. For example, Figure 1 uses data for Medicare beneficiaries of all ages. Had the data been restricted to Medicare beneficiaries 80 years of age or older, the chart might have given quite a different impression.

We frequently see charts or graphs that are misleading because their zero base is omitted. Compare, in Figure 2, the impression made by Chart A, which shows the number of deaths from firearms by year but without a zero reference point, with Chart B, which contains an appropriate zero reference.

Chart A creates the impression that the number of deaths declined sharply from 1979 to 1983. In Chart B, however, this same change appears as only a small variation in the typical levels experienced annually. What downward trend may exist appears small relative to the absolute level of firearm deaths.

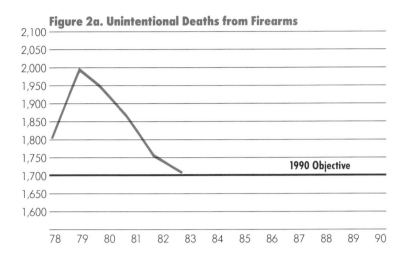

Figure 2a. Unintentional Deaths from Firearms

1990 Objective

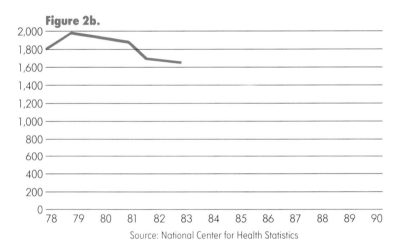

Figure 2b.

Source: National Center for Health Statistics

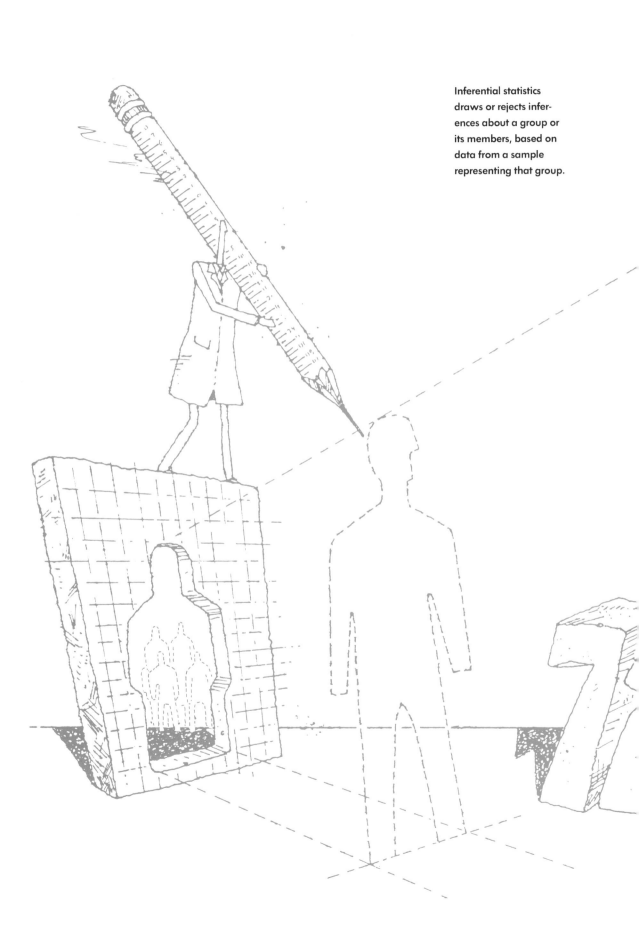

Inferential statistics draws or rejects inferences about a group or its members, based on data from a sample representing that group.

Inferential
Statistics

nferential statistics draws or rejects inferences about a group or its members, based on data from a sample representing that group.

We are all familiar with the colloquial use of the term *probability,* its derivatives, and related words: "You probably will be on your feet in a few days." "It is unlikely that this medicine will have any side effects." "The chances of recovery after this operation are good."

Probability

In each case, the terms *probable, likely*, and *chances* refer to probability.

Although most people would be hard pressed to give a precise definition of *probability,* most tend to assume that, if something is "probable," we can expect it will happen more often than not. This is actually quite a good working definition of probability.

Still, the study of probability has gone much further than this. Since it first arose at the gaming tables in Paris (where gamblers developed rules to help them determine how to place bets), probability has been refined, given a formal mathematical basis, and applied to many different fields.

Among these is inferential statistics, to which it is central. No discussion of inferential statistics would be complete, or even possible, without an examination of probability.

To understand this subject better, it is helpful to go back to its roots in gaming, and also helpful to look at a relatively simple game, such as tossing a coin. Like many events, a coin toss contains an inherent tendency toward variation: Because the coin has two sides, the coin can land either heads or tails, and probably will not always land the same side up every time it is tossed.

Probability is the means by which such variation may be quantified and thus made easier to express. It is typically expressed as a fraction between 0 and 1, or the corresponding ratio, decimal, or percentage. If you toss a coin in the air, the probability that it will land heads up is expressed by saying that it is "one-half"—or "one in two," ".50," or "50 percent."

As long as an event takes place in an unbiased environment (for instance, the coin isn't weighted so that it always lands heads up), it can be relatively easy to calculate the probability that the event will have a specific outcome. The probability can be calculated as a ratio of the number of ways an event can have a specific outcome to the number of ways it can happen in any way at all: A coin has only one head, but it can land one of two ways—heads up or tails up. Thus, the probability that the coin will land heads up is one in two.

A roulette wheel provides a slightly more complicated example. It has a total of 38 numbers, of which 18 are red, 18 are black, and two are green. If the wheel is "fair"—if nothing is done to bias the way it acts—the probability that the ball will fall into a black slot is exactly 18 (the number of black slots) in 38 (the total number of slots), or 9/19, or .4737, or 47.37 percent.

When an event occurs in such a way that the results are not known in advance but can be described entirely in terms of probability— we say that it is *random* or that it takes place *according to chance*. The toss of a coin is random; the probability of a head is one-half.

In a series of random events, the outcome of one event will not affect the outcome of another. Thus, for example, each time we toss a coin there is a 50 percent probability that it will land heads up. If the coin is tossed a second time this probability is not altered. The coin does not remember what happened on the previous throw.

If we were to toss the coin many times, probability does indicate that 50 percent of our coins should land heads up. But this is an idealization of what would actually happen if we tossed the coin. In practice, while it is likely that the coin would land heads up 50 times out of 100 throws, it might actually land heads up 20 times or 60 times—any number of times. There is even a real, though admittedly unlikely, possibility that 100 percent of the coins we tossed would land heads up.

Generally speaking, the more times an event takes place, the more likely it is that—overall—the outcomes of all the repetitions will eventually conform to probability. Thus, if we were to toss a coin thousands of times and kept a record of each toss, we could ultimately expect to find that—again, overall—50 percent of the time the coin had landed heads up. For each toss, however, the probability of landing heads up would continue to be only 50 percent.

Naturally, it is far easier to establish probabilities for the behavior of coins and roulette wheels than for many other events in which there is inherent variation. It is relatively easy to insulate such "games of chance" from influences that might bias the results. In contrast, most events that are subject to variation—from weather to the behavior of human beings—are subject to many influences other than chance.

Nevertheless, it is possible, and frequently necessary, to establish probabilities for complex events such as human behavior. Typically this is done by making an empirical observation of a sample of the larger population for which probabilities are to be established. The probability is calculated as the ratio between the number of times the specified outcome is achieved and the number of times the event actually occurred. The probability that is found in the sample population is assumed to apply equally to individual members of the population as a whole.

For example, let's say we observed that 73 percent of a sample of patients with the flu were able to resume normal activity within three days. Under appropriate circumstances, we might be able to infer a 73 percent probability that any individual with the flu will resume normal activity within three days.

The probability of 73 percent is an *unconditional* probability applicable to the population as a whole. Naturally, if we were in possession of more information, such as the age of the patient, we might well say that the probability of his resuming normal activity within three days is other than 73 percent. The probability that a given flu sufferer will resume normal activity within three days, knowing that he is over 75 years old, may be only 38 percent. Such a probability is called *conditional*—conditional on the patient's age being greater than 75.

The more information we have, the more we can divide a group as a whole into subgroups to which conditional probabilities can be assigned, and the more accurate we can make our probability statements about individual members of these subgroups.

Frequently it is impossible, impractical, or completely uneconomic to obtain data about every member of a population. We cannot, for example, survey every individual who ever has had or ever will have the flu, any more than we can chart the course of all thunderstorms.

Sampling

If we wish to know more about such populations, then, it becomes necessary for us to derive our information from a sample group. Inferential statistics is the science by which we create such a sample, then derive inferences that will be valid for the group as a whole.

Statistical sampling is used frequently in our society: Political polls are based on samples of voters; television ratings are based on samples of households with television sets. The Health Care Financing Administration uses a sample consisting of 5 percent of Medicare claims in order to obtain a wide variety of statistics relating to the basis for and magnitude of Medicare payments. The Food and Drug Administration samples foods and drugs in order to insure that they meet prescribed standards of purity and cleanliness. Peer Review Organizations sample hospital admissions and diagnoses in order to monitor quality of care.

The procedure typically used to create a sample is as follows:

Define the Underlying Population

We first define the underlying population to be represented. In some cases the underlying population can, without great difficulty, be placed on some list or array in which every member of the population is included. For example, the list of all physicians having an active license in the state of Illinois could be obtained from the licensure board in the state. On the other hand, the underlying population may consist of entities that—for any of a variety of reasons—cannot be listed. For example, it would be impractical, if not impossible, to obtain a list of all laboratory tests of urine for glucose.

Regardless of whether we can list all the members of our population, we must ensure that membership in the underlying population is precisely defined: If the underlying population is to consist of physicians licensed in Illinois, are we concerned only with physicians holding MD degrees or are DOs also included? Are we concerned about those licensed in the state of Illinois or those practicing in the state of Illinois? What constitutes practice?

Choose a Sampling Frame

From this information we construct a *sampling frame*, a means by which to give each member of the underlying population a known probability of being selected into the sample. If our underlying population consists of Illinois MDs, for example, the sampling frame may consist of a list acquired from the Illinois licensure board, consisting of every physician who is a member of the underlying group.

Sometimes the sampling frame must be constructed in two stages. If our underlying population consists of all laboratory tests of urine for glucose, for example, we first identify all licensed laboratories, and append to this list laboratories operated within hospitals and by physicians, which are not separately licensed. This gives us a primary sample, which is designed to be as complete as possible under the circumstances. We then draw on the logs kept by these laboratories to create a list of all urine tests for glucose that have been conducted by the laboratories in our primary sample.

Select the Sample

Having chosen a sampling frame, we may now select the members of the sample—a process that must be designed so that it does not introduce bias into the selection process. Another way to put this is to say that the process by which members of a sample are selected must be random.

Random selection is frequently achieved by a procedure comparable to spinning a roulette wheel, only the slots on the wheel are numbered to correspond to members of the underlying population. With each spin of the wheel, we note the number of the member at which the wheel stops, and that individual is drawn into the sample. In practice, of course, we are unlikely to use a wheel: Typically, an equivalent procedure is implemented by computer.

Stratified Samples

The examples given thus far have been examples of what is known as *simple* or *undifferentiated samples*. However, it can be shown theoretically, and is intuitively obvious, that a *stratified sample* may be more useful in some situations than an undifferentiated sample would be.

To draw a stratified sample we first define the strata into which the underlying population will be divided. These strata should cover the entire population and be defined, to the extent possible, by characteristics that may show a relationship with the data to be collected from the sample.

For example, in order to elicit data about physician fees in a state, we might stratify the physician population by size of the community in which the physician practices and, within the community, by physician specialty.

After the strata are defined, each stratum is represented by a separate sampling frame. We then choose members at random from each.

Estimation is one of the ways that inferential statistics draws inferences about a group or its members based on data from a sample representing that group. It refers to the process whereby we study the sample group, then draw inferences about the characteristics of the group as a whole.

In medicine, it is often necessary to draw conclusions about a larger group by studying a sample of that group. For example, morbidity rates, the proportion of a specified population with a specific disease, are frequently obtained by making estimates based on a sample of the population. This is particularly true for diseases other than the reportable communicable and venereal diseases.

Another common use of estimation in medicine is in judging the effectiveness of a drug. Obviously, we cannot "test" a drug in a population consisting of all patients to whom the drug might be prescribed in the future. Of necessity, an estimate of the drug's effectiveness will be drawn from a sample of patients.

Point Estimates

We have already discussed (pages 13 to 15) that data derived from an appropriate sample may be used to formulate a statement of the probability that a given event will have a specific outcome. For example, let's say that Drug A is shown to be effective in 80 percent of a sample group of patients with Diagnosis X. Under appropriate circumstances we may then say that there is an 80 percent probability that any person with this diagnosis, to whom Drug A is administered, will recover.

As we also discussed, this statement of probability further indicates a strong likelihood that Drug A would be effective in 80 percent of the underlying population from which our sample was drawn. This would be particularly likely if we were looking at the overall result of administering the drug to large numbers of people. Thus, we may estimate that Drug A would be effective in 80 percent of people with Diagnosis X.

Estimates such as this one, given in the form of a single, specific number, are referred to as *point estimates*. Examples include, "The mean length of stay is 3.7 days," "Drug A has been found effective for 80 percent of the population with Diagnosis X," or "The susceptibility of pre-school children to Disease Y is 24 per thousand children."

Yet, as we have also discussed (again pages 13 to 15), it is by no means certain that a point estimate will be consistent for any sample of the population to which it is applied: Drug A would not necessarily be effective in 80 percent of any group of people with Diagnosis X. In practice, there will be variation in the drug's rate of effectiveness from sample to sample.

For this reason it is common to accompany a point estimate with a statement about how closely we expect our estimate to mirror the data we would derive if we conducted successive samples of the population. This statement is made in terms of high and low points within which we believe that the relevant characteristic (or characteristics) of the population would fall.

When the estimate is an arithmetic mean, we may state a *standard error.* E.g., "The sample mean of 3.7 days has a standard error of 1.4 days." (The standard error is calculated as the standard deviation of the data divided by the square root of the sample size.)

Interval Estimates

Another way to state an estimate about data that can be expected to vary in practice is to make what is known as an *interval estimate.* To make such an estimate, we establish a range—from low point to high point—that is associated with some percentage of the population. Any percentage may be used, although the percentages most often found in the literature are 95 percent and 99 percent.

Interval estimates corresponding to point estimates given above would be as follows: "Ninety-five percent of the population is expected to have a length of stay ranging from 3.1 days to 4.8 days." "If Drug A is administered to a group of patients with Diagnosis X, it may be expected to be effective in from 73 percent to 84 percent of these patients." "If we were to take repeated samples in order to estimate the susceptibility of children to Disease Y, 99 percent of the time our estimates would be between 19 per thousand and 30 per thousand."

We may also state a probability (a *confidence coefficient*) that the relevant characteristic(s) of the underlying population would fall within a *confidence interval.* The confidence interval can be a range: e.g., "With confidence of 95 percent, Drug A would be effective for a percentage of the population falling within the range of 75 percent to 85 percent." The confidence interval can also be an interval above and below the sample mean: e.g., "With confidence of 95 percent, the mean of the population would fall within 2.8 units above or below the sample mean."

One way in which interval estimates are frequently used in medicine is in assessing a laboratory reading, such as the measure of serum cholesterol. We estimate that about 50 percent of the population of American white males aged 45-69 has a total serum cholesterol falling in the range (195,240) mg/dl. Ninety percent have a reading in the range (160,275). The range associated with 95 percent of the population is frequently termed *normal*. (The normal range, of course, is not necessarily associated with good health.)

As a rule, if the percentage chosen is small, the range it is associated with will be narrower than it would be if the percentage were larger. However, the increase in the range will not necessarily be proportional to the increase in the percentage. This is because, in many populations, some members will have results much above or well below the range that typifies the majority of the population. We may determine, for example, that 95 percent of the population of adult males has a diastolic blood pressure (mm Hg) between 66 and 107. But to include 99 percent of the population, the range might have to be widened to 58-119.

Statisticians consider interval estimates to be more useful than point estimates in most situations; thus interval estimates are often used in preference to point estimates.

Inferential statistics also draws inferences by formulating a hypothesis concerning an entire group, then testing this hypothesis by studying a sample of that group.

Testing Hypotheses

Hypothesis testing is often used when we wish to compare one group to another—for example, to compare patients treated with a new drug with patients treated with one already in use, to compare the length of stay of patients in one hospital with that of patients in another, or to compare the results of a procedure performed by one physician with the results of the same procedure performed by other physicians within a community.

In order to demonstrate the procedure by which a hypothesis is tested, let's say we wish to compare the length of stay experience for patients of Doctor A with that of other patients admitted to the same hospital for diagnosis-related group (DRG) 127. Doctor A has 18 patients whose mean length of stay is 10.2 days, with a standard deviation of 6.1. There are 87 other patients, whose mean length of stay is 7.9 days with a standard deviation of 5.7.

The problem: to determine whether the differences between Doctor A's patients and the others tell us anything significant about the care being provided by Doctor A.

How do we make this determination? First, before we can compare any two groups, it is essential to assure that they are comparable except for the characteristic to be examined—in this case, the quality of care they have received. Thus we must be able to assume that two groups of patients in this example are comparable in terms of such critical characteristics as age and history. It would not be valid to compare Doctor A's patients with other patients in the same hospital if, for example, Doctor A's patients were significantly older than the other patients.

We now formulate a hypothesis: "The mean length of stay for

Doctor A's patients admitted under DRG 127 is the same as that of other patients in the same hospital." The hypothesis to be tested is called the *null hypothesis*. It is essential that this hypothesis be stated unambiguously.

Next we state an alternate hypothesis. This is the hypothesis that will be accepted if the null hypothesis is rejected; conversely, it will be rejected if the null hypothesis is accepted.

The alternate hypothesis can be stated in more than one way— e.g., "The mean length of stay of Doctor A's patients is different from that of the other patients," or "The mean length of stay of Doctor A's patients exceeds that of the other patients." The difference between these statements of the alternate hypothesis is important because it affects the statistical calculations that follow and thus the inferences to be drawn.

If we ultimately reject the null hypothesis, we will never be absolutely certain that our decision was the correct one. Thus we must now state a *level of significance:* This is the probability we are willing to tolerate that we may have incorrectly rejected the null hypothesis. The level of significance is often symbolized by $[\alpha]$, the Greek lower case alpha.

The level of significance is not set based on statistical criteria. The decision is essentially a subjective one, which should be based on a careful consideration of the consequences of an incorrect decision. In our example, we might ask the following: What are the consequences if we incorrectly conclude that the length of stay of Doctor A's patients differs from that of other patients? What are the consequences to Doctor A? To the community? Will there be any monetary effect, and if so what? Answers to these and other such questions will guide us in setting the level of significance for this test.

The level of significance is usually set at a small value—frequently at 5 percent, which many people accept as reasonable. But there is nothing magic about this number. There is no reason why, under special circumstances, it might not make sense to set the value at 1 percent, which is usually considered conservative, or 2 percent or, alternately, at 20 percent.

We must now calculate the *observed probability* of accepting the null hypothesis often symbolized by p. This is the probability that, if the null hypothesis were valid, the difference between the two groups in our test would be as large as or greater than it in fact was. In other words, we are calculating the probability that the difference we observe between the two groups is due to chance.

In pursuing our example, we ask the following: Assuming that there is no difference between Doctor A's patients and other patients, what is the probability that the observed differences between the two groups would be as large as it is or even larger?

The calculation of observed probability can be quite complex, and typically will require reference to *statistical models,* which are discussed in the following chapter (pages 21 to 30). The calculation of observed probability for this test is thus provided in an appendix (pages 58 to 59). Suffice it to say here that the value of p will differ depending on the alternate hypothesis we have chosen.

Ultimately, if the observed probability exceeds the level of significance (mathematically, this is stated, "If p>α"), we accept the null hypothesis. Conversely, if the observed probability is less than or equal to the level of significance (p≤α), we reject the null hypothesis and accept the alternate.

In our example, if p>α, we conclude that whatever differences we may have observed between Doctor A's patients and other patients are not statistically significant; another way to express this is to say that they could have been caused by chance. If p<α, we accept the appropriate alternative hypothesis—either that the length of stay of Doctor A's patients differs from that of other patients or that the lengths of stay of Doctor A's patients are longer than those of other patients.

Each time a coin is tossed, there is a probability of 50 percent that it will land heads up. This is referred to as a *constant probability* governing this event.

Yet, as we have seen (pages 13 to 15), each toss of the coin is independent of each other throw. Thus it is at least possible that the coin could land heads up 20 times out of 100, or 60, or even 100.

The outcomes of "real world" events typically show great variation. And yet there is a pattern underlying this variation. By making countless empirical observations of events such as tossing coins, statisticians have discovered that the "real world" can often be described in terms of certain observed probabilities—different from the constant probability, although derived from it.

For example, if we toss a coin thousands of times, it is most likely that the coin will land heads up 50 percent of the time. It is still less likely that the coin would land heads up only 5 percent of the time, or 95 percent. Furthermore, specific probabilities can be assigned to these outcomes.

In short, variation in the "real world" can often be described in terms of specific observed probabilities. Statistics attempts to reflect this underlying pattern through what are called *statistical models*—idealized statements of the observed probabilities governing events when they are actually carried out. Statistical models are idealized representations of practical situations.

Such models are extremely useful. For example, we know that the constant probability governing the toss of a coin is 50 percent. But that in itself tells us very little about how often the coin would actually land heads up exactly 50 times in 100 throws. However, using a statistical model, we can calculate the probability of getting "heads" 50 times (or 10 times, or 75 times) within 100 throws.

Statistical models play an important role in statistics: They enable us to assign probabilities to a specific outcome of a chosen event, to confidence intervals, and to hypotheses.

A statistical model is generally written in the form of a mathematical equation. However, each statistical model can also be represented by a *curve* plotted on two axes, one of which (typically the y axis) is a sequence of probabilities. On the other axis (typically the x axis), is plotted the actual outcomes possible to an event. (In statistics, what we are here calling an *event* will typically be referred to as a *variable*, and its outcome will be referred to as its *value*.) These values, in turn, are calculated as a product of one or more *parameters*.

Statisticians have created a variety of statistical models to describe different types of events. Each statistical model produces a different class of curves.

Binomial Distribution

Consider first a very simple case in which an event has two possible outcomes. We might call these "success" and "failure," "zero" and "one," or "positive" and "negative." It can refer to any other complementary dichotomous conditions—such as a patient's response to a given drug, or whether an individual will become ill from a specified disease during a calendar year. An outcome of this type is called a *binomial variable*.

To consider a concrete situation, let us assume that the event we are attempting to describe consists of tossing two dice. If the face value of the dice totals seven, we characterize the toss as a success, otherwise a failure. As is well known to those who play with dice, the probability of a success—i.e. tossing a seven—is 1/6 and the probability of a failure is 5/6. (We could, of course, just as easily be discussing an emergency room in which there is a one-in-six probability that any given patient will be admitted to the hospital on any given night.)

Imagine that we toss the two dice 100 times. In terms of the

Figure 3. Number of Actual Outcomes with Specified Number of Sevens (150 Repetitions of 100 Tosses of Two Dice)

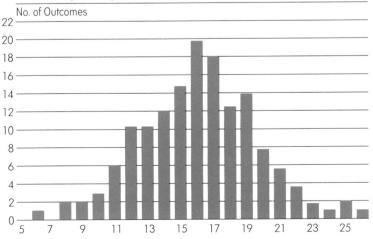

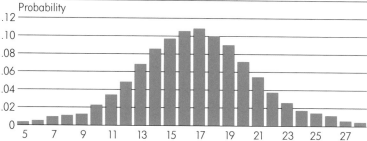

Figure 4. Theoretical Probability of Obtaining a Specified Number of Sevens (100 Tosses of Two Dice)

constant probability alone we might expect 16.67 successes out of the 100 tosses. However, this is not necessarily what would happen in practice. For one thing, of course, we cannot get a partial success. Furthermore, in practice, dice have no memory and no conscience: They do not "know" how they landed on previous throws. Each throw being governed by probability independent of all the others, it is even possible—however unlikely—that we could throw nothing but sevens.

The bar chart in Figure 3 shows the actual number of successes obtained in 150 repetitions of 100 tosses of the dice.

As this chart demonstrates, on one occasion, the dice added up to seven only six times out of 100. On another occasion, the dice added up to seven 26 times out of 100. Of all the sets of 100 throws, the greatest number—19—resulted in 16 "successful" throws of the dice. And the second greatest number—18—resulted in 17 successful throws.

Thousands upon thousands of empirical observations such as these have helped us to formulate a law called the *binomial distribution*. It gives us an idealized picture of the probability of achieving a specific outcome when that outcome can be expressed as a binomial variable (e.g., a successful throw of the dice). The parameters that determine this outcome (the binomial variable) are the constant probability (in our example, 1/6) and the number of times the event is repeated.

The binomial distribution can be represented by a curve that resembles the curve created by the bar chart above, but in idealized form. For 100 throws of the dice, this idealized distribution is depicted in Figure 4.

An idealized curve such as the one in Figure 4 provides a great deal of information about the theoretical probabilities associated with an event: It shows us, for example, that in 100 tosses of two dice there is a theoretical probability of slightly more than 10 percent that we will throw seven 17 times. We can also use the curve to determine the probability of throwing a number of sevens within a certain number of repetitions: i.e., by adding the probabilities associated with throwing 10 sevens and all lesser numbers of sevens, we discover that the probability is about 4 percent of obtaining 10 or fewer sevens in 100 throws of the dice—highly unlikely, but possible.

We could also, if we wished, compare the results we achieved using real dice with this idealized distribution, in order to determine whether we were using "fair" dice. Thus, if we really did throw seven 100 times in a row, we might well suspect—though we could not prove—that we were using crooked dice.

Normal Distribution

In some situations, an event results not in success or failure but in an actual number—such as a length of stay in the hospital, the increase in weight of a baby in the second three months of life, or the number of red blood cells per cubic millimeter in a sample of blood.

Here, the parameters that will be used to calculate the probability of different outcomes are the standard deviation (usually designated by the Greek letter sigma μ) and the arithmetic mean (usually designated by the Greek letter σ).

The most important statistical model of this type is the familiar bell-shaped curve known as the normal or *Gaussian distribution*. An important characteristic of the normal distribution is that 95 percent of the outcomes lie within 1.96 standard deviations on either side of the mean. In such distributions, the curve is *symmetrical*— each tail of the curve is equidistant from the central point, which corresponds with the mean. (Thus, for a normal distribution, the mean is also the median.)

The heights of adults tend to produce a distribution that is symmetrical in shape and will closely approximate a normal distribution as depicted in Figure 5.

A normal distribution can be derived even from data that, originally, were not normal. By taking successive random samples of these data, we can calculate a succession of means. The distribution of the mean values will closely approximate a normal distribution.

One important use of the normal distribution is to assess the probability of a specific outcome under the assumption that a hypothesis is valid, as mentioned on pages 19 to 21. The hypothesis is evaluated by a distribution, commonly a normal distribution, such as the one in Figure 6.

The arrow represents the observed outcome of an individual

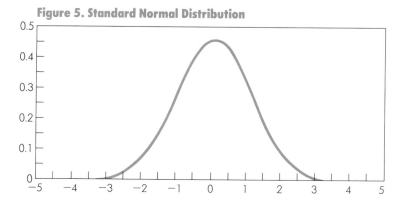

Figure 5. Standard Normal Distribution

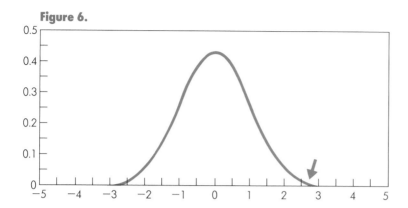

Figure 6.

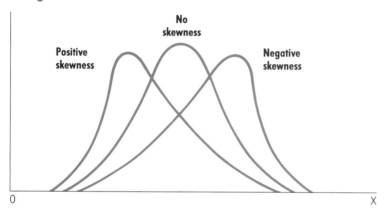

Figure 7. Skewed Distributions

No skewness

Positive skewness

Negative skewness

0   X

experience—possibly a patient's length of stay or total hospital bill. The curve represents the distribution of comparable outcomes as predicted by the null hypothesis. If the individual outcome is close to the mean of the distribution—i.e., the outcome associated with a high probability—we can say that the individual outcome is not inconsistent with the hypothesis. However, if the arrow is at one of the tails of the distribution—as is shown in the example—we can conclude that this event is very unlikely if the null hypothesis is valid. Depending on the level of significance we have chosen, we might then reject the null hypothesis and opt for the alternate hypothesis instead.

Non-Normal Distributions

The same parameters that produce a normal distribution may also produce a curve that is *skewed* (that is, not symmetrical). Curves may be skewed positively if the range of possible outcomes on one side of the mean is larger than the range of outcomes below the mean, negatively if the reverse is true. Figure 7 provides examples of negatively and positively skewed curves.

An example of a skewed curve is one depicting the distribution of the weight of the adult population: The curve is skewed positively

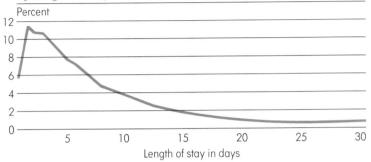

Figure 8. Distribution of Live Prospective Payment System Discharges for All Diagnosis-Related Groups, Calendar year 1984, by Length of Stay

because there are many more people weighing more than the mean than there are people who weigh less than the mean.

Another example is the distribution of incomes, which is skewed because some individuals have incomes that far exceed the mean with no counterpart of people whose incomes are far less than the mean. Yet another example is the results of laboratory tests such as serum bilirubin and creatinine, where the mean is very close to zero but there is a large interval possible above the mean.

Many events that take place in the "real world" do not conform to a normal distribution. Take, for example, the length of stay of live Medicare discharges for all DRGs combined, as shown in Figure 8. The arithmetic mean is 7.6 days, and the standard deviation is 7.0 days.

Lengths of stay below zero are impossible, so that the curve is skewed to the right. Furthermore, the left edge does not come down to zero, but remains significantly above zero because a sizable number of patients leave during the first day.

The diversity of distribution shapes for different DRGs can be appreciated by comparing as in Figure 9, the distribution of length of stay for DRG 148 (major small and large bowel procedures, age over 69 and/or complicating conditions) with DRG 410 (chemotherapy).

Poisson Distribution

The *Poisson distribution* characterizes the frequency with which an outcome of low probability takes place. Examples include the number of deaths per day in a hospital and the number of fatal motor vehicle accidents in a given geographical area per week. The historical illustration most often given in the statistical literature is the frequency with which a soldier in the Prussian Army was killed by being kicked by a horse.

The illustration in Figure 10 represents the Poisson distribution characterizing the number of times per week a fatal automobile accident occurs, assuming that the arithmetic mean of the number of accidents occurring per week is one.

The Poisson distribution demonstrates the relative frequency with

Figure 9a. Distribution of Live Prospective Pricing System Discharges for DRG 148, Calendar year 1984, by Length of Stay

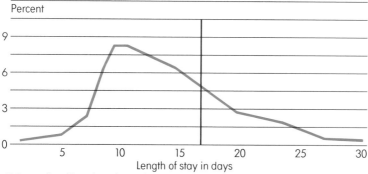

Percent

Length of stay in days

[1]Major small and large bowel procedures, age over 69 and/or complicating conditions.
Note: Vertical reference line is geometric mean as published in *Federal Register*, September 1, 1983

Figure 9b. Distribution of Live Prospective Pricing System Discharges for DRG 410, Calendar year 1984, by Length of Stay

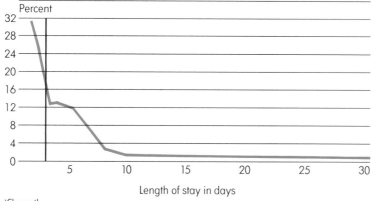

Percent

Length of stay in days

[1]Chemotherapy
Note: Vertical reference line is geometric mean as published in *Federal Register*, September 1, 1983

Figure 10. Poisson Distribution with Mean Equal to One

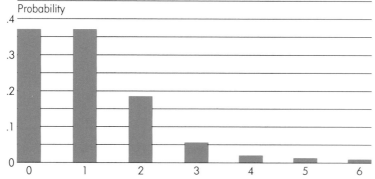

Probability

which we can expect zero accidents, one accident, two accidents, and so on within a given week. It shows, for example, that the probability of one accident and of zero accidents is the same. There is a relatively high—though lesser—probability of two, three, or even more accidents in one week. There is a probability of one in 1,000 that there would be six or more accidents in one week.

The Poisson distribution is governed by only one parameter, its mean value. This would be the one statistic worth knowing if we were trying, for example, to evaluate the impact of a mandatory seat belt law.

Derived Distributions

Many distributions have been defined in the statistical literature and have been used to characterize different types of data. Two are encountered relatively frequently in analyses of the results of experiments: These are the *t-distribution* and the *chi-square distribution*, which is usually denoted by the Greek letter [x^2].

Both of these distributions have their mathematical roots in the normal distribution—which, in fact, can be said to underlie much statistical theory.

t-distribution. When plotted as in Figure 11, the t-distribution looks like a normal distribution but with somewhat longer tails.

This distribution, often called the *Student's distribution* or *Student's t*, is used to determine the length of a confidence interval or to measure the probability of a hypothesis being valid in cases where we must estimate the standard deviation from a sample.

The shape of a t-distribution is dependent upon a single parameter called the *degrees of freedom*, frequently denoted by the Greek letter nu (v). The number of degrees of freedom is the number of data points—that is, the size of the sample—less the number of parameters that have been estimated from the data.

Figure 11. Comparison of Normal Distribution and "Student" *t*-distribution

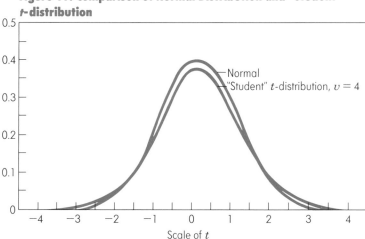

Measuring Medical Practice

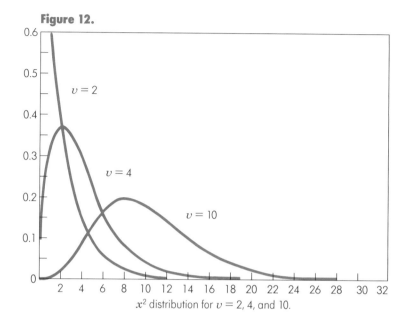

Figure 12.

x^2 distribution for $v = 2, 4,$ and 10.

In most cases, the number of degrees of freedom is one less than the size of the sample because the mean has been estimated.

The larger the sample size, the more closely the t-distribution will approximate a corresponding normal distribution. For most practical purposes, if the number of degrees of freedom is 30 or more, the t-distribution is indistinguishable from a normal distribution. For clinical evaluation this is highly desirable.

x^2 distribution. The x^2 distribution is most often used in instances where one wishes to determine whether observed outcomes are different from those expected. It is derived from a normal distribution by considering the distribution of the sum of squares of normally distributed variables that have a zero mean and whose standard deviation is 1. The x^2 distribution allows no negative values because it is the sum of squares. It is also characterized by a single parameter, also termed the degrees of freedom, which is equivalent to the number of independent quantities being squared and added together. The shapes of x^2 distributions for varying numbers of degrees of freedom are shown in Figure 12.

As the number of degrees of freedom increases, the distribution becomes more and more symmetrical.

The x^2 distribution is used to determine the confidence intervals for standard deviations and to test the equivalence of two sets of data.

Regression

Regression analysis is a way of expressing the relationship between one variable—described as *dependent*—and one or more other variables, which are described as *independent.*

For example, a nutritional study of 39 countries attempted to determine the relationship between the age-adjusted death rate per 100,000 population (the dependent variable) and levels of animal fat in the diet (the independent variable). It was discovered that, on average, the death rate increased by 1.6 per 100,000 for each 10 grams of animal fat added to the diet. This relationship can be expressed by the following equation, or *regression line:*

y = 2.5 + 0.16x

where y is the age-adjusted death rate per 100,000 and x is the average daily animal fat intake in gm/day.

Regression analysis attempts to find the equation that, in some sense, best describes the data. Many techniques may be used to determine an equation that fits the data. The one most often used is called the *least squares criterion*—i.e., the equation which minimizes the sum of the squares of the difference between the dependent variable as observed and that predicted by the equation.

Most regression problems include not one but many independent variables. One purpose of such analysis is to determine whether the relationship between the dependent variable and an independent variable is statistically significant and, if so, the magnitude of the relationship.

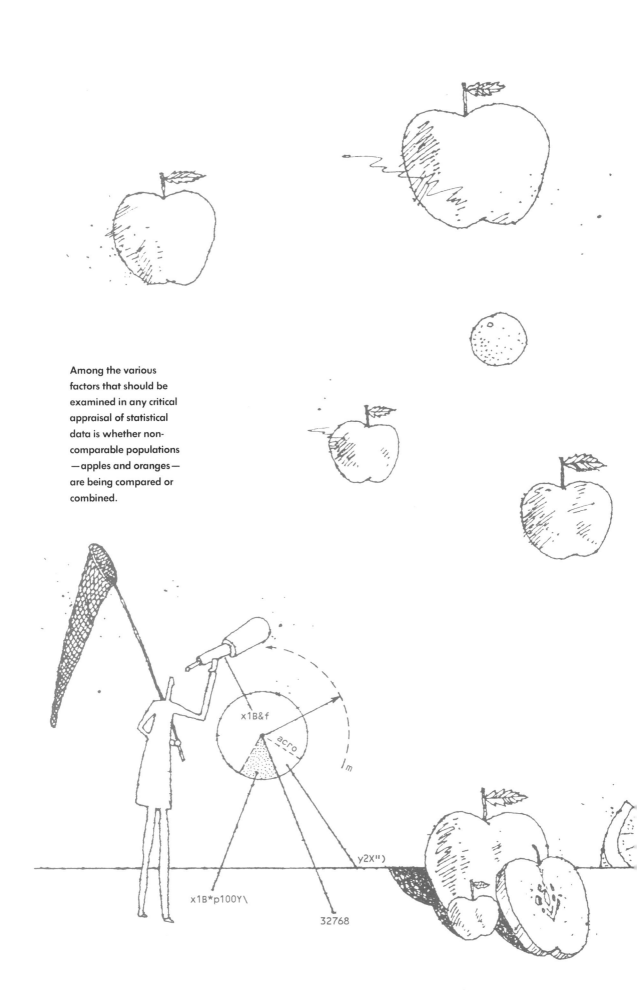

Among the various factors that should be examined in any critical appraisal of statistical data is whether non-comparable populations —apples and oranges— are being compared or combined.

x1B&f

acro

m

y2X")

x1B*p100Y\

32768

Assessing
Statistical Data

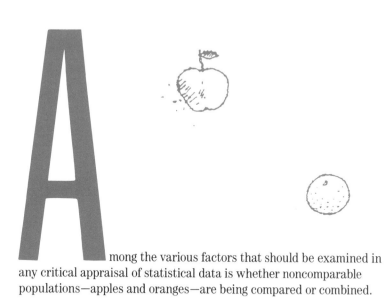

Among the various factors that should be examined in any critical appraisal of statistical data is whether noncomparable populations—apples and oranges—are being compared or combined.

**Noncomparable
Populations**

Comparing Noncomparable Populations

This booklet has already discussed (pages 15 to 17) the necessity of constructing a precise definition of the underlying population about which inferences will be drawn. An extension of this principle, which has also been alluded to earlier (pages 19 to 21), is that data about an individual or population can be compared only with data from a population that is known to be similar in all respects other than the one characteristic to be studied.

For example, we should not compare fees charged by rural family practitioners for certain surgical procedures with the fees charged by specialists in major metropolitan centers for the same procedures. So, too, the statistics that describe events in small voluntary hospitals may be very different from otherwise comparable data taken from major teaching hospitals, because the underlying patient mix is often very different.

Noncomparable populations are sometimes inadvertently compared because of unsuspected differences in the instruments with which the data were collected. For example, let's say that we wished to determine differences in attitudes between people living on the East and West coasts. Differences in the way survey questions were phrased, or even the types of people who conducted the interviews, could mean that the survey results would not actually reflect the differences we had set out to study.

Likewise, scientists must take special care if data to be compared are produced in different laboratories: The instruments in both laboratories must be regularly and carefully calibrated against a common standard, so as to ensure that the results from the two labs are comparable.

Combining Noncomparable Populations

Another potential problem in statistics is that of drawing an invalid inference from data that have been derived by combining noncomparable populations.

In order to illustrate this problem, let us assume that we are attempting to assess the effectiveness of an experimental drug ("A") by comparing it with a drug already in use ("B"). The following table shows the results obtained (in terms of deaths and recoveries) with both Drug A and Drug B in populations of 1,000 patients each.

	Recovered	Died	Total
Drug A	360	640	1,000
Drug B	560	440	1,000

The table shows that 36 percent of the patients receiving Drug A recovered, compared to 56 percent of those receiving Drug B. It appears obvious that Drug A is not more effective than Drug B. But is this really true?

In fact, these data were obtained by combining data collected at two hospitals. Perhaps the patient mix at the two hospitals was quite different. Certainly, the two populations appear to have been noncomparable.

In Hospital X the data were as follows:

	Recovered	Died	Total
Drug A	90	10	100
Drug B	540	360	900

Thus, at Hospital X, Drug A was 90 percent effective in a group of 100 patients, while Drug B was only 60 percent effective in a population of 900.

At Hospital Y, the data were as follows:

	Recovered	Died	Total
Drug A	270	630	900
Drug B	20	80	100

Here, 30 percent of 900 patients receiving Drug A recovered, while only 20 percent of 100 patients receiving Drug B recovered.

Obviously, in each of the two hospitals in which Drug A was tested, it outperformed Drug B. Yet when the numbers were combined, Drug B appeared to have outperformed Drug A.

Although this example is somewhat contrived, it demonstrates that, when we review any statistical analysis, we must be sure that the populations underlying any sample are clearly specified, so as to insure that noncomparable groups are not being combined.

Sampling is often employed informally in everyday life. We go to a restaurant and, on the basis of one or two experiences with the food there, characterize the culinary quality and the service. We travel to a foreign country and draw inferences about the friendliness of the citizens of that country based upon a sample of encounters with the local inhabitants. A patient's perceptions about a clinic are colored by a receptionist's behavior.

Inappropriate Sampling

Yet it is easy to see, from these examples, that inferences drawn from a sample need not necessarily be valid. A restaurant customer who eats only fish may not realize that a restaurant's beef dishes are excellent; a single encounter with a few Londoners will not give a valid picture of all English people. Inferences drawn from samples will be valid only if the sample group is appropriate.

Biased Sampling

One example of inappropriate sampling was the massive public opinion poll conducted by *Literary Digest* magazine during the 1936 presidential election, which predicted a sizable victory by Alf Landon over Franklin D. Roosevelt. The magazine made two errors that resulted in this invalid inference:

1. As its sampling frame, the magazine chose lists of people with telephones. However, many people at that time did not have telephones, and so were excluded. Being less well-off, people without telephones were more apt to be supporters of Roosevelt, the Democrat, than supporters of the Republican Landon. Thus the sampling frame chosen by the magazine did not adequately represent the underlying population, which consisted of all persons who were going to vote in the election.

2. The magazine sent out millions of ballots, but the individuals who received these ballots were free to decide for themselves whether to return them. This created *selection bias* in that the ballots tended to be returned by individuals who felt strongly about that election. Typically, those wishing a change are more likely to take an activist role, and this again favored the Republicans.

The *Literary Digest's* experience illustrates two ways in which it is possible to create an inappropriate sample:

1. We could choose a sampling frame that does not actually represent the population we are concerned about. For example, we could not obtain a valid sample of all physicians in a state by walking up to individuals in a hotel lobby at the state medical convention. A sample frame that included only physicians attending the state medical meeting might not represent all those practicing in the state.

2. We could select members of our sample in a non-random way. In the example just given, if the interviewer is given the latitude to determine whom to interview, he might be inclined to speak to physicians who struck him as more "approachable." Thus dress and other subjective factors might affect his selection, rendering it non-random.

There are a variety of other ways in which bias may be introduced into the selection of a sample. One is the use of volunteers: People who volunteer to provide information or participate in a study may not be representative of a population that includes people who did not and perhaps would not volunteer. Bias may even be introduced through the timing of a sample: The attitudes of people who have just woken up may not be representative of attitudes that would be found in the population as a whole; some laboratory results are likely to be different at different times of the day.

People cannot ordinarily be required to respond to a survey, and so survey results are often based on the responses of volunteers. As a result, surveys present a severe potential for biased sampling. Well-designed surveys attempt to overcome this problem in several ways, including making special attempts to reach potential respondents who did not immediately volunteer the requested information. In addition, various adjustments may be made in order to make the sample conform more closely with known characteristics of the underlying population: For example, if 32 percent of physicians who respond to a survey are family practitioners and it is known that family practitioners actually constitute 54 percent of the underlying population, the sampled responses can be weighted by the fraction 54/32. Likewise, physicians who are not family practitioners, who comprise 68 percent of the sample but only 46 percent of the population, would be given the weight 46/68. A similar result can be achieved through appropriate use of stratified samples (pages 15 to 17).

Naturally, any known bias in a sample should be taken into consideration if this sample is to be compared with another population. For example, if Drug A was tested on volunteers, we should be reluctant to compare its effectiveness with that of Drug B as revealed by hospital medical records. We might, however, create comparable populations by testing both Drug A and Drug B on volunteers.

Inadequate Sample Size

We can draw inferences from samples of any size, yet in general the smaller the sample the less credence can be given to the inferences drawn from it. We know intuitively that a single receptionist cannot adequately represent the staff of an entire clinic. And we have seen statistical models (pages 21 to 30) demonstrating that the fewer times an event is repeated the less likelihood there is that the outcome will conform to the constant probability.

Here is another example to illustrate the same point: Suppose that we wished to judge the effectiveness of one drug ("A") by comparing it with another ("B"). Drug B is known to be effective for 50 percent of patients. Drug A is tested in a group of patients and found to be effective in 80 percent of cases. We decide to compute the probability that we would have achieved the same result (in the group of patients on whom Drug A was tested) if we had administered Drug B.

If this were an example of hypothesis testing, we would now undertake a formal procedure, such as we have described earlier (pages 19 to 21). In order to make our point about the importance of sample size, however, we need make only a couple of relatively simple calculations.

Let's say that Drug A was tested on a very small group: only five patients … of whom four (80 percent) showed improvement. How probable is it that we could have achieved the same result using Drug B? Take the probability that the drug will be effective in each patient: 50 percent. Multiply that figure by itself once for each patient in the sample: 50 percent x 50 percent x 50 percent x 50 percent x 50 percent = 3.125 percent. Multiply this figure by five, which is the number of ways a 4:1 split can be obtained from five patients: 6.25 percent x 5 = 15.63 percent. There is a 15.63 percent probability that Drug B would be effective in four out of five cases. This is a relatively high level of probability, given that the level of significance is typically set at 5 percent. Thus, at best, we can say only that we are not persuaded Drug A is more effective than Drug B.

But say that we test Drug A again, on 100 patients. Once again it is effective in 80 percent of cases. The probability that Drug B would be effective for 80 patients out of 100 is only about one in one hundred thousand (00.001 percent). At this level, the probability is quite low, a convincing indication that the 80 percent effectiveness rate of Drug A is a significant improvement over the effectiveness of Drug B.

Sample size can be especially critical when the data drawn from the sample are expressed as percentages. A small sample will tend to yield very large, potentially misleading, percentages: Thus, if one of two children has the flu, we may say that 50 percent of the population has the flu; others might find this statistic quite impressive if they did not know the size of the sample on which it was based. Yet a percentage drawn from a small sample will change dramatically as a result of a relatively small change in the underlying data: If the second of our two children develops the flu, our percentage immediately increases to 100 percent.

In contrast, if one out of 100 children had the flu, only 1 percent of our population would be ill. If one more child became ill, the percentage of children with the flu would increase only to 2 percent.

Another major source of incorrect inferences in statistics is the use of procedures predicated upon invalid assumptions.

Invalid Assumptions

Many procedures in common use assume a normal distribution of the data; however, data are not typically normal. In many cases, the data may be sufficiently non-normal so that inferences drawn on the assumption of normality will be invalid. We have seen, for example, (pages 21 to 30) that length-of-stay data for Medicare DRGs are typically non-normal. Any procedure assuming normal distribution should be applied to such data with great caution.

The use of procedures based upon the binomial distribution may be invalid if assumptions made about the parameters underlying that distribution are invalid. For example, a probability that has been assumed to be constant—applying to all the events in the distribution— might not be the same for all repetitions of the event. In order to achieve a constant probability, the outcome of each repetition of an event, such as the tossing of a coin or the examination of a patient, should be independent of every other outcome. But the outcomes may not be independent of one another. For example, examinations performed on siblings may not be unrelated in their outcomes if one child has an infectious disease.

Inappropriate Use of Statistical Inferences

Even if statistical methodologies are themselves impeccable, inferences drawn from them may yet be used inappropriately. A particular danger is the tendency to assume that statistics are capable of *proving* an inference.

As we have seen throughout this booklet, inferential statistics makes statements about probabilities. At most, based on statistics, we can say only that a particular outcome is highly probable or highly improbable. We cannot assure that a particular outcome will take place. Nor can we prove causation with statistics: e.g., we cannot prove statistically that a pair of dice are loaded or that a given population of patients are receiving inadequate medical care.

The testing of hypotheses is particularly fraught with the danger that a hypothesis found *probable* will be assumed to have been *proved*. This is never a valid assumption, for the following reasons:

First, it must always be remembered that the statement of null and alternate hypotheses and the specification of the level of significance are not statistical decisions. The hypotheses are chosen based on the nature of the investigation, and the level of significance is chosen based on the protection desired or needed against the possibility of falsely rejecting the null hypothesis. The statistical contribution is in the methodology, which incorporates these non-statistical specifications to reach an inference.

Second, hypothesis testing does not allow us to reach conclusions with complete certainty. If the level of significance for a test were set at 5 percent, for example, we would still expect that, one time in 20, the analysis would lead us to incorrectly reject the null hypothesis. Like estimation, hypothesis testing makes statements about probabilities, not certainties.

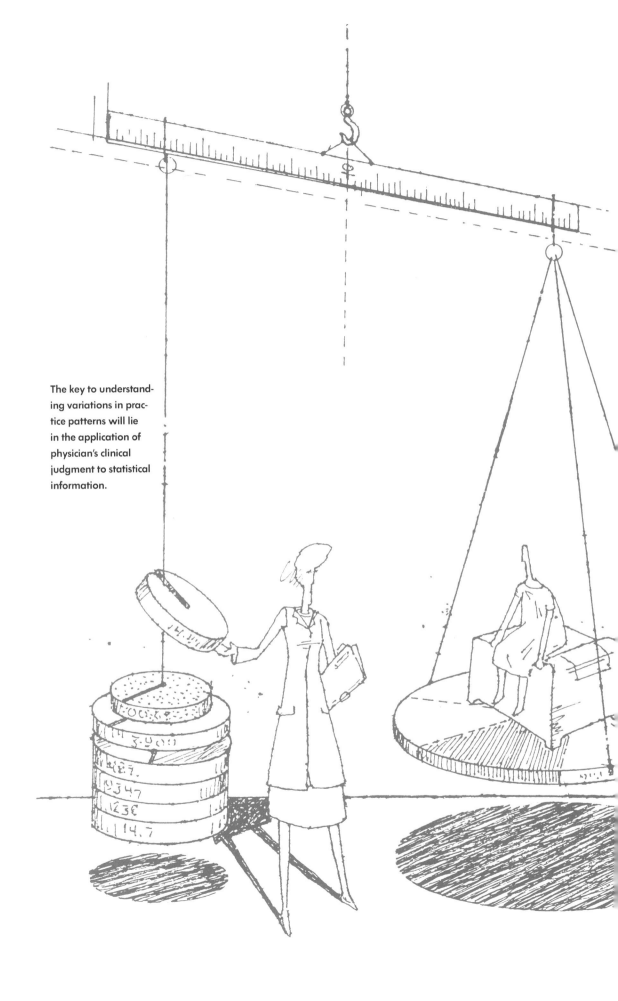

The key to understanding variations in practice patterns will lie in the application of physician's clinical judgment to statistical information.

Statistics and
Health Policy Issues

The following chapters present some current examples of health policy issues for which physicians will likely encounter data and statistics in their medical practices. Selected examples include: variations in utilization of health care services; hospital mortality data; and utilization review, quality assurance and peer review.

Since the importance of these issues will likely increase in the coming years, it is essential that physicians understand the appropriate role of statistics in their evaluation. This is particularly true in those instances (e.g., release of hospital mortality data) where physicians may be called on by patients to explain the clinical meaning of published data. Hopefully, the information presented in the preceding chapters will provide a solid foundation upon which appropriate evaluation of these data can be based.

Hospital Mortality Data

The Health Care Financing Administration (HCFA), which administers the Medicare program, is currently planning to release selected statistical information on the performance of those hospitals which participated in the Medicare program in 1986.

The information to be released would include, for each hospital, the number of Medicare beneficiaries treated and the percentage of beneficiaries who died within 30 days of admission. This information is to be compared with an estimate of the number of deaths that would be expected at the same hospital (calculated through a regression analysis) if that hospital's experience conformed to the national experience with patients of similar age, sex, incidence of complicating diseases, and prior hospitalization in 1986. HCFA has taken the position that a comparison of data drawn from the individual hospital with the estimate drawn from the population as a whole will give consumers useful information about the quality of care provided by individual hospitals.

Release of such data can, of course, have important implications. As such, it is essential that any information not be misleading to the public. However, as may be inferred from the previous chapters, there is at least one fundamental flaw in the design of this plan which may foster the proliferation of misleading statistics: In essence, the HCFA plan invites reviewers of these data to compare noncomparable populations (see pages 33 to 35).

The population that is subject to comparison consists of Medicare beneficiaries with a specific diagnosis in a hospital. Given the plan proposed by HCFA, the population to which comparisons will be made may differ from this population in several important ways. These include the following:

1. *Race.* In drawing an estimate from the overall population, HCFA has ignored race as a factor that could influence the outcome of specific procedures. Thus a hospital that, because of location, has a preponderance of patients who are of one race may be compared with a hospital population that serves several races.

2. *Medicare status.* While each hospital's data are drawn from Medicare patients alone, the national population of citizens over the age of 65 includes people who are not on Medicare. Medicare covers those with prior social security coverage and their dependents. It does not include those who did not work, or who did not work in a covered occupation, such as federal employees without other jobs. In addition, while Medicare does cover some individuals under age 65, such as those with end-stage renal disease, these individuals are not comparable to members of the population as a whole who are in the same age group.

3. *Severity of illness.* No measure of the severity of illness is included in the estimate drawn from the national population. As a result, a hospital that may selectively receive patients whose condition is more critical, or that receives more terminally ill patients, will inevitably show mortality rates higher than those estimated.

Because of these deficiencies, questions have been raised about whether the methods being used by HCFA can produce valid predictions of mortality rates for specific hospitals. It has further been questioned as to whether it is appropriate to imply that differences between a hospital's mortality rate and an estimated national mortality rate are due solely to the quality of care provided by the hospital. The number of factors that could influence such an outcome (i.e., the mortality experience) is simply too great to permit inferences to be drawn about any one factor.

Indications are that HCFA will release these data in December 1987, most likely in a format demonstrated in Figure 13. This Figure helps illustrate some of the interpretation problems that may arise. The limitations of the data, of course, center on outliers—cases where the actual mortality rate falls outside the range of predicted mortality rates. These data lead one to believe that there may be a quality problem whenever the actual mortality rate is above the upper end of the range of predicted mortality rate.

The key question that must be addressed is the reasons that

Figure 13. Sample Hospital Mortality Data

Diagnostic Category		Cases	Actual Mortality Rate (%)	Range of Predicted Mortality Rates (%)
All Causes		1028	18	11 to 18
CA	Cancer	34	32	14 to 45
CE	Cerebrovascular Accidents	62	39	18 to 42
GC	Gastrointestinal Catastrophes	28	39	6 to 35
GI	Gastrointestinal Disease	153	5	2 to 11
GU	Urologic Disease	45	4	1 to 19
GY	Gynecologic Disease	7	8	0 to 100
HL	Low-Risk Heart Disease	116	2	2 to 10
HM	Severe Chronic Heart Disease	46	33	12 to 56
HS	Severe Acute Heart Disease	57	48	28 to 35
ME	Metabolic/Electrolyte Disturbances	54	22	18 to 35
OP	Orthopedic Disorders	18	6	0 to 31
PU	Pulmonary Disease	152	32	15 to 30
RU	Renal Disease	30	47	14 to 52
SE	Sepsis	17	29	18 to 53
TR	Trauma	18	11	1 to 33

any such outlier might occur. An example is the diagnostic category "HS—severe acute heart disease." The actual rate shown of 48% is above that predicted, 28 to 35%. This outlier could occur for several reasons including:

1. The normal random error that is expected in any statistical model. Some observations always lie above the regression line;

2. The exclusion of important explanatory variables from the predictive model (e.g., severity of illness, race, Medicare status of the hospital); and

3. A quality problem may actually exist in this diagnostic category in this hospital.

The problem is that there is no easy way for the public to discern which of the reasons is the correct one. Accordingly, it is essential that physicians understand, and be able to inform their patients, as to what can be legitimately inferred from these data.

Geographic Variations in the Utilization of Health Care Services

A substantial and growing body of research has identified significant differences from one geographic area to another in the utilization of health care services. For example, tonsillectomies have been found to vary from 151 per 10,000 population in one area to as few as 13 per 10,000 in another. Hysterectomies have been found to be performed on 70 percent of women in one locality compared to 30 percent in another.

A key issue raised by these data is whether these differences in utilization can be explained by demographic or epidemiologic factors. (In other words, are these populations comparable?) Are there a greater number of elderly in one area than in another, for example? Is it possible that individuals requiring certain types of treatment are being referred from one geographic area into another? Statistical research indicates that often such area-to-area differences cannot be explained solely in terms of demographic or epidemiologic differences. Any number of other factors (e.g., variations in patient needs, differences in medical practice styles) may be important.

Figure 14. Maine Laminectomy Rates, 1984

Area	Observed	Expected	OBS-Exp	O/E Ratio
1	45	26	+19***	1.70
2	58	36	+22***	1.63
3	172	109	+63***	1.58
4	27	19	+8	1.39
5	21	17	+4	1.25
6	95	79	+16	1.20
7	34	30	+4	1.13
8	32	29	+3	1.12
9	16	15	+1	1.09
10	17	17	0	1.02
11	67	68	−1	.98
12	51	52	−1	.98
13	43	44	−1	.98
14	26	29	−3	.91
15	16	28	−12	.90
16	196	220	−24	.89
17	22	26	−4	.84
18	92	115	−23*	.80
19	12	16	−4	.77
20	47	62	−15	.76
21	11	16	−5	.71
22	19	28	−9	.69
23	12	18	−6	.67
24	9	14	−5	.63
25	10	16	−6	.62
26	10	17	−7	.58
27	7	18	−11*	.40
28	6	15	−9*	.39
29	4	11	−7	.37
30	4	12	−8*	.35
State Total: 1,181		1202	0	1.00

Source: Maine Medical Assessment Program, 1987

*=95% Confidence Level; **=99%; ***=99.9%

Another issue raised by such variations is whether certain health care services are being provided unnecessarily in some areas of the country. Simply because in one area there is a relatively high incidence of a specific procedure, it cannot be assumed that the procedure is being performed unnecessarily. It is equally possible that in an area with a relatively low rate of a given procedure, the procedure may not be performed often enough. Too little provision of medical services is as undesirable as too much.

The Maine Medical Assessment Program

One of the most comprehensive studies to review statewide variation rates in utilization is the Maine Medical Assessment Program (MMAP), initiated under the auspices of the Maine Medical Association in 1981. The MMAP, composed of an advisory committee that includes individual physicians and representatives of the insurance industry, hospital groups and state agencies, reviews hospital discharge data and identifies variations in specific medical and surgical procedures among the states' 31 hospital market areas. Additionally, specialty-specific study groups of physicians, each headed by a specialty group representative from the advisory committee, look closely upon a course of action to educate physicians identified as statistical "outliers" to the problem area. This educational, peer review process of the study groups is important in the development of a consensus about the appropriateness of utilization patterns.

An example of an issue recently approached by the MMAP was substantial variation in the laminectomy rate across the state's hospital market areas for 1,181 such procedures performed in 1984. (These rates are shown in Figure 14.) After viewing the charted data, the advisory committee believed the variations evident in statewide rates deserved special attention and a special study group of orthopedic and neurosurgeons was assembled.

Before these physicians saw the laminectomy information, prepared by the Maine Health Information Center, physician investigators ran the data through a final check to ensure that they were:

☐ credible (i.e., clinical, meaningful)

☐ timely (i.e., current, up-to-date); and

☐ that they would be presented in a manner to help educate the physicians to "outliers" in their respective hospital market areas.

When the study group met to review the laminectomy rates, investigators asked each physician first for an assessment—a definition—of his own standard of medical care for the procedure. All of the responses, not surprisingly, were comparable. Each member felt he used a conservative approach to surgery.

The group was then asked to perform an informal, retrospective review—a medical audit—of medical records from high, medium and low rate areas to determine if even rudimentary outcome measures were available from patient records. Four orthopedists agreed to provide records of their own patients for analysis. Each physician reviewed the records of the others, recording prescribed information on type and duration of symptoms, type and findings of clinical tests, precise operative procedure and apparent outcome.

Although a formal review of surgical incidences has not been completed (and with the goals of the program in mind, review will be an ongoing process), the study group did not advocate a plan to reduce the incidence of high rates of surgery in the state. The group instead determined that educating physicians to variations in the procedure and studying outcome results more closely "would be of significant value in reducing this specific variation." Other similar medical procedures are scheduled for investigation.

Utilization studies are stimulating a re-evaluation of medical practice patterns around the United States, an assessment that is certain to have a major, long-term impact on both the cost and the quality of health care. However, it is evident that variations in practice patterns cannot be understood on the basis of statistics alone. The impact of these variations must be weighed—not only on health care costs but also on patient welfare. Ultimately, the key to understanding these variations will lie in the application of the physicians' clinical judgment to statistical information.

As the Maine experience has demonstrated, the benefits of a regional variations study may extend far beyond the program's interpretation and discussion of hospital discharge data. An equally valid purpose is in the educational process of bringing practice variations and their meanings to the attention of physicians.

Utilization Review, Quality Assurance, and Peer Review

The application of statistical concepts to medical practice data is a major component of utilization review and quality assurance processes. There is likely to be increasing use of such statistical applications in these areas, due to the greater amount of medical care data being generated by payment systems, and due to the increasingly sophisticated techniques for evaluating and comparing such data.

Nearly all medical review programs make use of the same statistical principles discussed earlier. For example, it is not at all uncommon for reviewing bodies to examine data that indicate specific hospitals or physicians who exhibit practice patterns that significantly deviate from the median level of care provided for a particular diagnosis. Such analysis can lead to the identification of utilization "outliers," i.e., hospitals or physicians who provide significantly more or less services to a particular kind of patient compared to other hospitals or physicians. The same analysis can be applied to mortality rates and other data that may be regarded as indicators of possible quality problems.

While definitive judgments concerning appropriate utilization and quality of care typically must await the review of the medical chart by a physician, a key component of review programs is the development of screening criteria that can be applied to all, or a sample, of cases as an administratively efficient means of detecting possible utilization or quality problems. Those flagged as possible problems can then be referred for further medical review to determine if a problem in fact exists.

The following sections describe some recent and emerging uses of extensive data analysis in medical review. These areas include:

☐ severity of illness measures;

☐ accreditation of health care organizations;

☐ peer review organizations (PROs); and

☐ private utilization review.

Severity of Illness Measures

In recent years there has been growing interest in the notion of "measuring quality." Researchers, as well as payors interested in obtaining maximum value for their health dollar, have explored a number of ways in which empirically-derived quantifiable indicators of the quality of medical care can be identified. One of the key components of quality assessment activities such as these is a mechanism for adjusting cases by the severity of illness of the patient on admission. This step is necessary because quality measurement systems use information contained on the patient medical record or insurance claim form indicating admitting diagnosis or disease category, yet there is a wide disparity in severity of illness among patients within a particular diagnosis or disease category. This disparity is often significant enough to distort outcome data which fails to take severity into account.

There are at least five leading systems used by hospitals to measure severity of illness that also are being used to assess quality of care. All of them employ to varying degrees the data and statistical analysis techniques discussed earlier. For example, MedisGroups, developed by MediQual Systems, classifies patients at admission on the basis of severity of illness derived from objective clinical findings. Computerized software integrates severity information with hospital resource use data (length of stay and charges) so that analysis can be undertaken of the care being performed at the individual physician level. Another system, Apache II (developed by William A. Knaus of the George Washington University Medical Center), assesses severity of illness of intensive care unit patients based on objective clinical criteria and then assigns an empirically-derived probability of death based on that severity level. A provider whose patterns of treatment reflects a higher than predicted death rate would be subjected to further investigation. The other systems are Patient Management Categories (PMC) developed by Wanda Young of the University of Pittsburgh; Disease Staging, developed by SysteMetrics, Inc.; and CSI, computerized severity index, developed by Susan Horn of Johns Hopkins University.

Accreditation

The Joint Commission on Accreditation of Healthcare Organizations is currently undertaking a major restructuring of its hospital accreditation process. The primary focus will shift from a periodic review of administrative structure and function to a continuing evaluation of clinical processes and outcomes. This revised evaluation process will have two major elements:

☐ Development by the Joint Commission and use by the hospital of (a) "clinical indicators" of quality health care which can be used as screening criteria to identify problem areas, and (b) "organizational indicators" which are those administrative and management activities believed to most directly affect quality of care.

☐ Expansion of the Joint Commission survey process to include continuous monitoring of the hospital's collection and use of these clinical and organizational indicators to improve quality, and feedback to the institution on its performance.

In effect, the Joint Commission will expand the basis of its accreditation decisions to ask not only "can this institution provide quality health care," but also "does it" provide such care. Plans call for pilot testing of the new survey process in early 1988, and an expanded on-site field trial with about 100 hospitals in 1989. Full implementation of a revised process for hospitals is projected for the early 1990's.

Peer Review Organizations

Utilization and Quality Control Peer Review Organizations, or PROs, are organizations under contract to HCFA to conduct review of care provided to Medicare beneficiaries. They review a 3% random sample of Medicare discharges, review all readmissions within 15 days of discharge, apply generic quality screens to cases they review, and make appropriate adjustments to DRG codes submitted by hospitals. In the current contract period, PROs are also obligated to focus on HCFA identified outliers, i.e., specific hospitals and physicians that the data indicate significantly deviate from median levels of care or mortality.

There are two general PRO activities that may impact on a physician: admission review/DRG validation, and quality review. In their current contracts and under recently enacted legislation, PROs are obligated to direct more of their resources to quality review. Specifically, under legislation enacted in 1986, PROs are required to undertake the following additional review responsibilities:

☐ To conduct quality review of HMO and competitive medical plan (CMP) services.

☐ To deny payment for care not meeting professional standards.

☐ To conduct 100% preadmission/preprocedure review of 10 surgical procedures.

☐ To review all, or at the discretion of the Secretary, a sample of ambulatory surgical procedures performed in ambulatory surgical centers and hospital outpatient departments.

▢ To review posthospital care rendered between an initial admission and readmission where the readmission occurs less than 31 days after the discharge. This review is to include a quality review of post-hospital services after the first admission in all settings, including skilled nursing facilities and home health agencies, except for care provided in physicians' offices.

▢ To assure that a reasonable proportion of a PRO's activities be in the review of quality of medical care, including post-hospital care and care rendered in ambulatory settings.

The result of an adverse PRO finding arising from admissions review is generally denial of payment for the Medicare service provided. The result of an adverse quality finding by a PRO could lead to consequences that are far more serious—the imposition of a sanction by the Inspector General of Health and Human Services which may be in the form of temporary exclusion from participation in the Medicare program.

Private Utilization Review

Utilization review programs conducted by hospitals may include certification of hospital stays, quality assurance activities and development of *physician profiles.* Physician profiles are of particular interest, as they are intended to chart a given physician's hospital practice patterns and compare these patterns to other physicians within the hospital. Ostensibly, the purpose of physician profiles is to assist physicians in determining if they are practicing "mainstream" medicine or if their practice patterns are radically outside the norm. Accordingly, physician profiles must be examined in light of the statistical caveats raised in the previous chapters.

For example, Figure 15 is a depiction of a physician profile which compares the age/sex, length of stay (LOS), mean LOS and total cost of pneumonia cases (DRG 89) for four different physicians. As demonstrated in Figure 15, the actual LOS of patients treated by physicians B, C, and D was under or very close to the national average mean LOS. Likewise, the total costs for provisions of care by the hospital was close to the DRG rate of reimbursement (i.e., hospital payment received) for DRG 89 in most cases. Physician A, however, treated patients who were hospitalized at least twice as long as the average LOS for DRG 89, and the cost for treatment of these cases far exceeded the DRG rate of reimbursement. However, before a utilization review activity concludes that physician A was overtreating patients or keeping them in the hospital too long, several key questions must be posed.

First, what are the characteristics of the group to which physician A is being compared? It is important to compare like groups or specialties if valid statements are to be made about practice patterns. For instance, if physician A is a sub-specialist and only treats the "worst cases" then it is logical to assume that the patients treated by physician A would require more intensive care and thus account for the

Figure 15. Sample Physician Profile

Physician	DRG	Sex/Age	Actual LOS	National Avg. LOS	Total Cost	DRG Payment
A	89	M-91	5	8.5	$ 5,705	$ 4,850
	89	F-77	30	8.5	$52,561	$ 4,850
	89	F-82	16	8.5	$16,992	$ 4,850
	89	F-89	15	8.5	$26,949	$ 4,850
B	89	F-79	7	8.5	$ 4,889	$ 4,850
	89	F-69	8	8.5	$ 7,510	$ 4,850
	89	M-78	7	8.5	$ 5,344	$ 4,850
	89	F-67	1	8.5	$ 1,263	$ 4,850
	89	F-75	3	8.5	$ 2,628	$ 4,850
C	89	F-63	3	8.5	$ 2,394	$ 4,850
	89	F-68	4	8.5	$ 3,804	$ 4,850
	89	F-73	3	8.5	$ 3,686	$ 4,850
	89	M-57	7	8.5	$ 3,598	$ 4,850
D	89	M-74	6	8.5	$ 3,452	$ 4,850
	89	F-67	2	8.5	$ 2,785	$ 4,850
	89	F-71	5	8.5	$ 3,978	$ 4,850
	89	M-73	8	8.5	$ 4,970	$ 4,850

higher total cost for care rendered.

Next, are physician A's patients different from the other physician's patients? That is, are the patients older, sicker, or do they have significant co-morbidities? As shown in Figure 15, physician A typically does treat older patients who may be more likely to have accompanying complications or co-morbidities, and thus contribute to a relatively long LOS.

Finally, do physician A's patients come from outside the normal catchment area for the hospital? Assuming that physician A was a sub-specialist, his patients may come from a larger catchment area which might include rural areas. Physician A may not have as readily available the option of discharging patients to home health services due to lack of appropriate facilities in the patient's home town. This may also contribute to a longer LOS.

In brief, before concluding that a physician is practicing outside the norms of medicine, a careful review of the statistical evidence must be conducted.

Corporations, third party payors, and other health delivery systems are also seeking to contain health care costs through various forms of utilization review. This review is in some ways similar to that conducted under the PRO program, but is performed either by non-government payors under contract to employers or by specialized "fourth party" review entities under contract to either the third party payor or directly to the employer. Examples of such private review activities include second opinion programs, pre-admission review, hospital stay certification, and discharge planning. Two of the most common of these approaches, second opinion programs and pre-admission review, warrant additional discussion.

Second opinion programs, often referred to as second surgical opinion programs, most commonly deal with the need for surgical intervention in an illness or injury. Such programs deal with situations where treatment can be deferred pending the reviewer's opinion without adding significantly to the problem the patient faces. Ordinarily, the second opinion is part of the patient's third party coverage and the insurer will recompense the physician who gives the second opinion for the examination. In some contracts, there may be a differential payment for the surgery in question between situations where the patient seeks a second opinion and those in which he does not. In programs where a second opinion is mandatory, the carrier will ordinarily not pay for recommended surgery unless there has been a second opinion. However, in most plans, the final decision as to surgery is left to the patient; even if the second opinion opposes surgery, the plan will pay for it if the patient decides to go ahead.

Preadmission review, a traditional feature of HMOs, is increasing as a utilization control procedure in the fee-for-service environment. The Blue Cross and Blue Shield Association, for example, estimates that 85 percent of the Blue Cross and/or Blue Shield Plans that underwrite hospital benefits offer some form of preadmission review (voluntary or mandatory), affecting anywhere from five to ten million individuals (out of the 77.5 million who are covered by their hospital insurance). In addition, many commercial insurers, self-insured employers, and state Medicaid programs have implemented some form of preadmission review.

In response to the demand for preadmission review programs, some 150 medical review organizations have appeared in the past several years to handle the administrative aspects of the programs. While the various organizations in the fragmented industry tend to share the same general philosophy regarding the desirability of reducing the level of inpatient hospital utilization, and while the "mechanics" of the preadmission review programs are often quite similar, the specific details and requirements of each program quite often differ significantly.

In some programs, only those physicians who have been determined to hospitalize patients at a higher than average rate are subject to preadmission review; in others, the focus is on specific procedures. In some programs, however, all admissions except emergencies are subject to review. In some cases, the burden appears to be on the patient to initiate the review process, in others it appears to be on the physician. In many programs though, it is unclear exactly where the responsibility lies. Also, depending on the specific program, various penalties can be imposed for failure to obtain preadmission approval, including partial or total nonpayment of a claim, even if an admission was medically necessary.

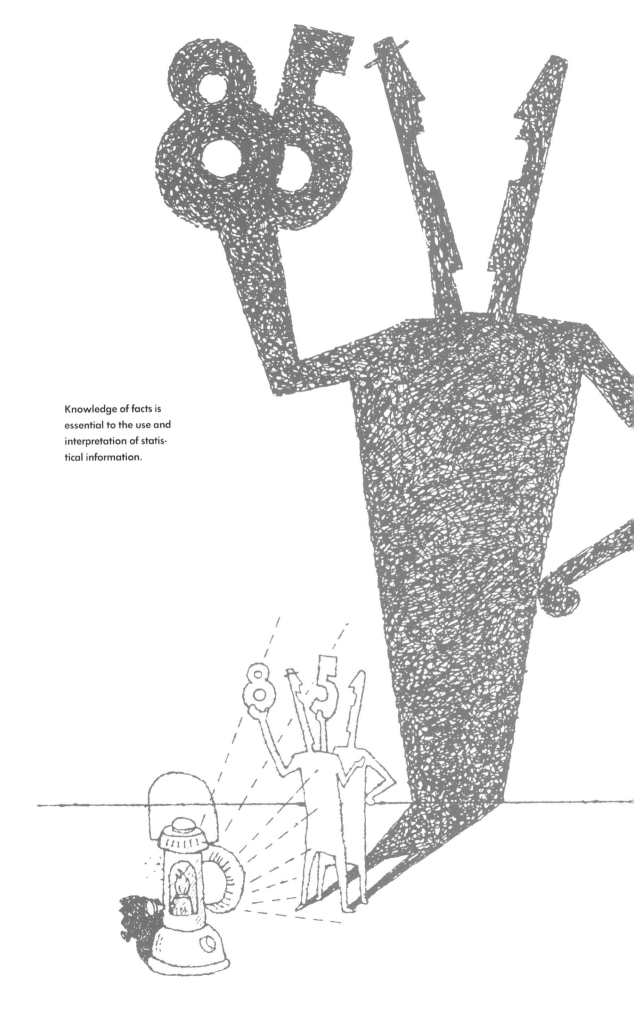

Knowledge of facts is
essential to the use and
interpretation of statis-
tical information.

Conclusion

If one message underlies much of what has been said in this booklet thus far, it is this: statistics is a tool—a useful, valuable tool. But it cannot be used in a vacuum. The inferences derived from statistics may not be appropriately interpreted in the absence of additional information.

Knowledge of facts is essential to the use and interpretation of statistical information.

By their very nature, statistics apply to groups; physicians treat individuals. For physicians this means that statistics are never—by any means—the whole story. Of equal or even greater importance are the medical factors to be considered. Nor should medical decisions ever be left to a statistician, even by default.

Nothing will substitute for the physician's knowledge of an individual's specific circumstances, or of biasing influences that may affect inferences drawn from a sample. Such knowledge may range from an awareness that board-certified specialists charge higher fees than other physicians do for certain procedures to an awareness of medical conditions that may affect an individual patient's response to a course of treatment.

Statistics is a tool, but only a tool. As is true of all tools, their worth depends on the hands that use them.

Glossary

Alternate hypothesis
The hypothesis to be accepted if the null hypothesis is rejected.

Arithmetic mean
A measure of central tendency calculated by summing all data values and dividing by the number of data values. Where no confusion may exist, also called the *average* or the *mean*.

B

Binomial distribution
A probability distribution that describes the frequency of occurrence of a set of outcomes as calculated by a constant probability and a specific number of repetitions.

C

Chi square distribution
A probability distribution determined by a non-negative outcome calculated using one parameter, the *degrees of freedom*.

Conditional probability
The probability under some qualifying assumption or condition.

Confidence coefficient
The probability that, in successive samples, a confidence interval constructed in a specified manner will include the specified outcome.

Confidence interval
An interval estimate whose likelihood of coverage of the specified outcome is equal to a specified confidence coefficient.

I

Interval estimate
An estimate of one or more outcomes expressed as a range of values expected to include the outcome(s).

L

Level of significance
The probability of incorrectly rejecting the null hypothesis in a test.

M

Median
That quantity in a set of data that is exceeded by half the data items and is itself as large or larger than half the data items. A measure of central tendency.

Mode
That quantity in a set of data that occurs more frequently than any other. The mode, a measure of central tendency, may not be unique.

N

Normal distribution
A probability distribution that assumes a symmetric bell-shaped curve. The normal distribution is determined by the mean and the standard deviation of the event in question.

Null hypothesis
The hypothesis to be tested.

P

Parameter
A quantity that may define the shape or location of a probability distribution, e.g., the mean.

Percentile
The p-th percentile in a set of data is that quantity which is larger than p percent of the data items and is exceeded by (100-p) percent. The 50th percentile is the median.

Point estimate
An estimate of an outcome expressed as a single number.

Poisson distribution
A probability distribution describing the frequency with which an event of low probability takes place. It is governed by one parameter, the mean value.

Population
The collection of all elements defined by some characteristic or set of characteristics. Elements may be people, objects, laboratory samples, or any definable set.

Probability
The likelihood of some event occurring, measured by a fraction between zero and one.

Probability distribution
A mathematical equation that provides the probability associated with each possible outcome of a specific event or with any interval covered by a continuous event.

R

Random
Described by a probability distribution.

S

Sample
A set of elements (people, objects, etc.) collected to represent some defined population.

Skewness
The lack of symmetry of a curve whereby one tail is longer than the other.

Standard deviation
A measure of the dispersion in a set of data that is equal to the square root of the mean value of the squares of the deviations of each data item from the arithmetic mean of that set of data.

Standard error
A measure of the dispersion of the arithmetic mean, a statistic calculated from a set of data. The standard error of a mean is equal to the standard deviation of the set of data divided by the square root of the sample size.

Statistic
A quantity calculated from a sample, e.g. the sample mean.

Stratified sample
A sample obtained by first dividing the underlying population into strata based on some defined characteristic(s) and then sampling within each stratum.

Symmetry
The property of curve where there exists some axis such that for each point on the curve to the right of the axis, there exists a point equidistant from the axis to the left.

T

t-distribution
A symmetric probability distribution with one parameter, the degrees of freedom.

Test of hypothesis
A statistical procedure that associates the probability of the consistency of obtaining an observed outcome with the assumption of the null hypothesis.

U

Universe
Synonym for "population."

Bibliography

American Medical Association, Dept. of Health Care Review, Division of Health Policy and Program Evaluation, *Confronting Regional Variations: The Maine Approach*, Chicago, 1986. Copies available from Order Dept., OP-007, American Medical Association, P.O. Box 10946, Chicago, Ill., 60610.

Paul Armitrage, *Statistical Methods in Medical Research*, New York, Wiley, 1971.

B. W. Brown and M. Hollander, *Statistics: A Biomedical Introduction*, New York, Wiley, 1977.

Theodore Colton, *Statistics in Medicine*, Boston, Little Brown, 1974.

W. Daniel, *Biostatistics: A Foundation for Analyses in the Health Sciences*, Third Edition, New York, Wiley, 1983.

A. Glantz, *Primer of Biostatistics*, New York, McGraw Hill, 1981.

A. B. Hill, *Principles of Medical Statistics*, Ninth Edition, New York, Oxford University Press, 1971.

G. Hoel, *Basic Statistics for the Health Sciences*, Palo Alto, CA, Mayfield Publishing Co., 1984.

A. Ingelfinger, *et. al. Biostatistics in Clinical Medicine*, Second Edition, New York, Macmillan, 1987.

E. Mathews and V. T. Farewell, *Using and Understanding Medical Statistics*, Basil, NY, Karger, 1985.

S. Levy and S. Lernshow, *Sampling for Health Professionals*, Belmont, CA, Lifetime Learning Publications, 1981.

J. N. Morris, *Uses of Epidemiology*, New York, Churchill Livingstone, 1975.

A. Murphy, *Biostatistics in Medicine*, Baltimore, Johns Hopkins University Press, 1982.

dH. Regier, *Biomedical Statistics with Computing*, Chichester, NY, Research Studies Press, 1982.

C. Schefler, *Statistics for Health Professionals*, Reading, MA, Addison-Wesley, 1984.

A. Sokal and F. Rohlf, *Biometry: The Principles and Practice of Statistics in Biological Research*, Second Edition, San Francisco, Freeman, 1981.

W. Turkey, *Exploratory Data Analysis*, Reading, MA, Addison-Wesley, 1977.

I. M. Weisbrot, *Statistics for the Clinical Laboratory*, Philadelphia, Lippincott, 1985.

Wonnecott and T. H. Wonnecott, *Introductory Statistics*, Fourth Edition, New York, Wiley, 1985.

Bill Williams, *A Sampler on Sampling*, New York, Wiley, 1978.

A Calculation
of Observed Probability
In Hypothesis Testing

The following calculation is provided so that the reader may, if desired, see the completion of a statistical analysis introduced earlier (page 19). This calculation also illustrates the use of statistical tables.

This is a calculation of observed probability, based on the same data that were used previously to illustrate hypothesis testing.

The problem is to compare the length of stay experience for Doctor A's patients with other patients admitted to the same hospital for DRG 127. The relevant statistical data are:

	Doctor A's patients	Other patients
Number (n)	18.0	87.0
Mean (x)	10.2	7.9
Standard Deviation(s)	6.1	5.7

We wish to test the null hypothesis "The mean length of stay for Doctor A's patients admitted under DRG 127 is the same as that of other patients in the same hospital." As the alternate hypothesis we can state "The mean length of stay of Doctor A's patients exceeds that of the other patients." We assume that the data have a reasonably normal distribution and set the level of significance to $2=.05$.

Our calculation of observed probability consists of evaluating

$$t = \frac{\overline{x}_1 - \overline{x}_2}{\sqrt{\dfrac{s_1^2}{n_1} + \dfrac{s_2^2}{n_2}}}$$

where the subscripts 1 and 2 refer to Doctor A's patients and all others respectively. By substituting, we obtain:

$$t = \frac{10.2 - 7.9}{\sqrt{\dfrac{(6.1)^2}{18} + \dfrac{(5.7)^2}{87}}}$$

$$\frac{2.3}{\sqrt{2.0672 + .3734}} \qquad \frac{2.3}{1.562}$$

$$= \qquad 1.4725$$

We refer to Table A of critical values of the t-distribution, now with $t = n_1 + n_2 - 2 = 103$ degrees of freedom. Interpolating vertically for 103 degrees of freedom, we see that t .90 = 1.2889 and t .95 = 1.6598. We can interpolate horizontally to approximate the percentile corresponding to 1.47 as follows:

Given:

Percentile	t
.95	1.6598
p	1.4725
.90	1.2889

then:

$$\frac{.95 - p}{.95 - .90} = \frac{1.6598 - 1.4725}{1.6598 - 1.2889}$$

$$\frac{.95 - p}{.05} = \frac{.1873}{.3709}$$

$$.95 - p = (.05)(.5050) = .0252$$

or:

$$p = .95 - .0252$$
$$= .925$$

approximately.

The probability that t would be greater than 1.4725 is $p = 1 - .925 = .075$. Thus, the observed probability is 7.5 percent of obtaining as large a difference between Doctor A's patients and others observed. Since this probability exceeds the level of significance, we do not reject the null hypothesis of equality of mean length-of-stay for Doctor A's patients and other patients.

Statistical
Tables

d.f.	$t_{.90}$	$t_{.95}$	$t_{.975}$	$t_{.99}$	$t_{.995}$
1	3.078	6.3138	12.706	31.821	63.657
2	1.886	2.9200	4.3027	6.965	9.9248
3	1.638	2.3534	3.1825	4.541	5.8409
4	1.533	2.1318	2.7764	3.747	4.6041
5	1.476	2.0150	2.5706	3.365	4.0321
6	1.440	1.9432	2.4469	3.143	3.7074
7	1.415	1.8946	2.3646	2.998	3.4995
8	1.397	1.8595	2.3060	2.896	3.3554
9	1.383	1.8331	2.2622	2.821	3.2498
10	1.372	1.8125	2.2281	2.764	3.1693
11	1.363	1.7959	2.2010	2.718	3.1058
12	1.356	1.7823	2.1788	2.681	3.0545
13	1.350	1.7709	2.1604	2.650	3.0123
14	1.345	1.7613	2.1448	2.624	2.9768
15	1.341	1.7530	2.1315	2.602	2.9467
16	1.337	1.7459	2.1199	2.583	2.9208
17	1.333	1.7396	2.1098	2.567	2.8982
18	1.330	1.7341	2.1009	2.552	2.8784
19	1.328	1.7291	2.0930	2.539	2.8609
20	1.325	1.7247	2.0860	2.528	2.8453
21	1.323	1.7207	2.0796	2.518	2.8314
22	1.321	1.7171	2.0739	2.508	2.8188
23	1.319	1.7139	2.0687	2.500	2.8073
24	1.318	1.7109	2.0639	2.492	2.7969
25	1.316	1.7081	2.0595	2.485	2.7874
26	1.315	1.7056	2.0555	2.479	2.7787
27	1.314	1.7033	2.0518	2.473	2.7707
28	1.313	1.7011	2.0484	2.467	2.7633
29	1.311	1.6991	2.0452	2.462	2.7564
30	1.310	1.6973	2.0423	2.457	2.7500
35	1.3062	1.6896	2.0301	2.438	2.7239
40	1.3031	1.6839	2.0211	2.423	2.7045
45	1.3007	1.6794	2.0141	2.412	2.6896
50	1.2987	1.6759	2.0086	2.403	2.6778
60	1.2959	1.6707	2.0003	2.390	2.6603
70	1.2938	1.6669	1.9945	2.381	2.6480
80	1.2922	1.6641	1.9901	2.374	2.6388
90	1.2910	1.6620	1.9867	2.368	2.6316
100	1.2901	1.6602	1.9840	2.364	2.6260
120	1.2887	1.6577	1.9799	2.358	2.6175
140	1.2876	1.6558	1.9771	2.353	2.6114
160	1.2869	1.6545	1.9749	2.350	2.6070
180	1.2863	1.6534	1.9733	2.347	2.6035
200	1.2858	1.6525	1.9719	2.345	2.6006
∞	1.282	1.645	1.96	2.326	2.576

Table A.
Percentiles of
the t-Distribution

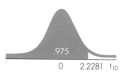

Source: W.W. Daniel, *Biostatistics: A Foundation for Analyses in the Health Sciences,*
Third Edition, New York, Wiley, 1983.

Table B.
Areas Under
the Standard Normal
Curve from 0 to z.

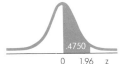

z	.00	.01	.02	.03	.04
.0	.0000	.0040	.0080	.0120	.0160
.1	.0398	.0438	.0478	.0517	.0557
.2	.0793	.0832	.0871	.0910	.0948
.3	.1179	.1217	.1255	.1293	.1331
.4	.1554	.1591	.1628	.1664	.1700
.5	.1915	.1950	.1985	.2019	.2054
.6	.2257	.2291	.2324	.2357	.2389
.7	.2580	.2611	.2642	.2673	.2704
.8	.2881	.2910	.2939	.2967	.2995
.9	.3159	.3186	.3212	.3238	.3264
1.0	.3413	.3438	.3461	.3485	.3508
1.1	.3643	.3665	.3686	.3708	.3729
1.2	.3849	.3869	.3888	.3907	.3925
1.3	.4032	.4049	.4066	.4082	.4099
1.4	.4192	.4207	.4222	.4236	.4251
1.5	.4332	.4345	.4357	.4370	.4382
1.6	.4452	.4463	.4474	.4484	.4495
1.7	.4554	.4564	.4573	.4582	.4591
1.8	.4641	.4649	.4656	.4664	.4671
1.9	.4713	.4719	.4726	.4732	.4738
2.0	.4772	.4778	.4783	.4788	.4793
2.1	.4821	.4826	.4830	.4834	.4838
2.2	.4861	.4864	.4868	.4871	.4875
2.3	.4893	.4896	.4898	.4901	.4904
2.4	.4918	.4920	.4922	.4925	.4927
2.5	.4938	.4940	.4941	.4943	.4945
2.6	.4953	.4955	.4956	.4957	.4959
2.7	.4965	.4966	.4967	.4968	.4969
2.8	.4974	.4975	.4976	.4977	.4977
2.9	.4981	.4982	.4982	.4983	.4984
3.0	.4987	.4987	.4987	.4988	.4988

.05	.06	.07	.08	.09
.0199	.0239	.0279	.0319	.0359
.0596	.0636	.0675	.0714	.0753
.0987	.1026	.1064	.1103	.1141
.1368	.1406	.1443	.1480	.1517
.1736	.1772	.1808	.1844	.1879
.2088	.2123	.2157	.2190	.2224
.2422	.2454	.2486	.2517	.2549
.2734	.2764	.2794	.2823	.2852
.3023	.3051	.3078	.3106	.3133
.3289	.3315	.3340	.3365	.3389
.3531	.3554	.3577	.3599	.3621
.3749	.3770	.3790	.3810	.3830
.3944	.3962	.3980	.3997	.4015
.4115	.4131	.4147	.4162	.4177
.4265	.4279	.4292	.4306	.4319
.4394	.4406	.4418	.4429	.4441
.4505	.4515	.4525	.4535	.4545
.4599	.4608	.4616	.4625	.4633
.4678	.4686	.4693	.4699	.4706
.4744	.4750	.4756	.4761	.4767
.4798	.4803	.4808	.4812	.4817
.4842	.4846	.4850	.4854	.4857
.4878	.4881	.4884	.4887	.4890
.4906	.4909	.4911	.4913	.4916
.4929	.4931	.4932	.4934	.4936
.4946	.4948	.4949	.4951	.4952
.4960	.4961	.4962	.4963	.4964
.4970	.4971	.4972	.4973	.4974
.4978	.4979	.4979	.4980	.4981
.4984	.4985	.4985	.4986	.4986
.4989	.4989	.4989	.4990	.4990

Source: W.W. Daniel, *Biostatistics: A Foundation for Analyses in the Health Sciences,*
Third Edition, New York, Wiley, 1983.

Table C. Percentiles of the Chi-Square Distribution

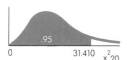

d.f.	$x^2_{.005}$	$x^2_{.025}$	$x^2_{.05}$	$x^2_{.90}$
1	.0000393	.000982	.00393	2.706
2	.0100	.0506	.103	4.605
3	.0717	.216	.352	6.251
4	.207	.484	.711	7.779
5	.412	.831	1.145	9.236
6	.676	1.237	1.635	10.645
7	.989	1.690	2.167	12.017
8	1.344	2.180	2.733	13.362
9	1.735	2.700	3.325	14.684
10	2.156	3.247	3.940	15.987
11	2.603	3.816	4.575	17.275
12	3.074	4.404	5.226	18.549
13	3.565	5.009	5.892	19.812
14	4.075	5.629	6.571	21.064
15	4.601	6.262	7.261	22.307
16	5.142	6.908	7.962	23.542
17	5.697	7.564	8.672	24.769
18	6.265	8.231	9.390	25.989
19	6.844	8.907	10.117	27.204
20	7.434	9.591	10.851	28.412
21	8.034	10.283	11.591	29.615
22	8.643	10.982	12.338	30.813
23	9.260	11.688	13.091	32.007
24	9.886	12.401	13.848	33.196
25	10.520	13.120	14.611	34.382
26	11.160	13.844	15.379	35.563
27	11.808	14.573	16.151	36.741
28	12.461	15.308	16.928	37.916
29	13.121	16.047	17.708	39.087
30	13.787	16.791	18.493	40.256
35	17.192	20.569	22.465	46.059
40	20.707	24.433	26.509	51.805
45	24.311	28.366	30.612	57.505
50	27.991	32.357	34.764	63.167
60	35.535	40.482	43.188	74.397
70	43.275	48.758	51.739	85.527
80	51.172	57.153	60.391	96.578
90	59.196	65.647	69.126	107.565
100	67.328	74.222	77.929	118.498

$x^2_{.95}$	$x^2_{.975}$	$x^2_{.99}$	$x^2_{.995}$
3.841	5.024	6.635	7.879
5.991	7.378	9.210	10.597
7.815	9.348	11.345	12.838
9.488	11.143	13.277	14.860
11.070	12.832	15.086	16.750
12.592	14.449	16.812	18.548
14.067	16.013	18.475	20.278
15.507	17.535	20.090	21.955
16.919	19.023	21.666	23.589
18.307	20.483	23.209	25.188
19.675	21.920	24.725	26.757
21.026	23.336	26.217	28.300
22.362	24.736	27.688	29.819
23.685	26.119	29.141	31.319
24.996	27.488	30.578	32.801
26.296	28.845	32.000	34.267
27.587	30.191	33.409	35.718
28.869	31.526	34.805	47.156
30.144	32.852	36.191	38.582
31.410	34.170	37.566	39.997
32.671	35.479	38.932	41.401
33.924	36.781	40.289	42.796
35.172	38.076	41.638	44.181
36.415	39.364	42.980	45.558
37.652	40.646	44.314	46.928
38.885	41.923	45.642	48.290
40.113	43.194	46.963	49.645
41.337	44.461	48.278	50.993
42.557	45.722	49.588	52.336
43.773	46.979	50.892	53.672
49.802	53.203	57.342	60.275
55.758	59.342	63.691	66.766
61.656	65.410	69.957	73.166
67.505	71.420	76.154	79.490
79.082	83.298	88.379	91.952
90.531	95.023	100.425	104.215
101.879	106.629	112.329	116.321
113.145	118.136	124.116	128.299
124.342	129.561	135.807	140.169

Source: W.W. Daniel, *Biostatistics: A Foundation for Analyses in the Health Sciences,* Third Edition, New York, Wiley, 1983.

Notes